The Pain of Surgical Operations before Anesthesia

Covering a previously unexplored area in the history of surgery, this innovative resource provides a historical overview of how surgeons managed the pain of an operation. The definitive statement on this book's central topic was written by Celsus in the first century AD, which emphasized accepting the unavoidability of pain during surgery and how patient distress should not tempt surgeons to rush procedures before completion. Inhaled narcotics were occasionally recommended but never became a standard treatment. There was a consensus from classical times that ingested opium produced too many side effects to be used during an operation. In 1846, anaesthesia was introduced, solving the problem.

Presenting these different eras in the history of surgery with a range of detailed examples, this book also offers inferential interpretations of how surgeons incorporated their understanding of pain into their surgical practice. Most surgeons demonstrated humanity, tempered by their beliefs and personalities, and managed pain by using specific techniques, instruments, and analgesic adjuncts.

Key Features:

- Provides an overview of an underexplored area of history, filling a gap in the history of medicine by focusing on pain during surgery before modern anaesthetics
- Offers inferential explanations for the ways in which surgeons managed pain prior to anaesthesia, including how they utilized specialized techniques and instruments, as well as how patients coped with pain when awake and unanaesthetized
- Builds a comprehensive understanding of the history of surgery prior to anaesthesia through historical examples and primary sources

With key topics, surgeons, and surgical techniques covered, this book will be suited to medical students taking courses on the history of surgery and will interest practitioners of various surgical specialties, anaesthetists, and medical historians.

The Pain of Surgical Operations before Anesthesia

Jeremy C. Ganz

CRC Press
Taylor & Francis Group
Boca Raton London New York

CRC Press is an imprint of the
Taylor & Francis Group, an **informa** business

Designed cover image: Getty Images

First edition published 2027
by CRC Press
2385 NW Executive Center Drive, Suite 320, Boca Raton FL 33431

and by CRC Press
4 Park Square, Milton Park, Abingdon, Oxon, OX14 4RN

CRC Press is an imprint of Taylor & Francis Group, LLC

ISBN: 978-1-041-25382-2 (hbk)
ISBN: 978-1-003-74881-6 (ebk)

DOI: 10.1201/9781003748816

Typeset in Times
by SPi Technologies India Pvt Ltd (Straive)

Dedication

Being a surgeon has this in common with being in the police: Only your colleagues can really understand the reality of your daily life. Since both professions include elements that are viewed with disfavour by those they serve, I should like to dedicate this book to my colleagues, past and present. We who have worked for a government-run health service know that dedication is a politician's excuse for paying less than the rate for the job. This dedication involves no such undercurrent. Inevitably, in such a complex field as surgery, opinions on optimal performance vary, and such opinions may be expressed with passion. I have met brilliant surgeons, less-gifted surgeons, and surgeons with whom I have passionately disagreed. Even so, the great majority of surgeons, and all of those whom I have met, have been engaged in doing their best for their patients, and it is to them that this book is dedicated.

Contents

Preface

This is a book about how surgeons and patients coped with the agony occasioned by a surgical operation prior to the invention of anaesthesia in 1846. The recording of clinical experience beyond mere observation and description began with Hippocrates, who died around 370 BC. The period from then to 1846 spans over two millennia. The period in which anaesthesia has been available is under two centuries. Thus, management of the pain of an operation has been a part of any surgical intervention for most of human history. It should be noted that a distinction is made between surgery and operations. In sport, matches take a relatively short time, while the entirety of the sport includes the much longer periods of training and practice. To consider operations as surgery would be the same as considering a sport to consist merely of matches: entertaining, perhaps, but incomplete.

John Bell of Edinburgh stated it very clearly:

> *Operations usurp an importance in surgical education which they should not naturally have (1).*

This book is not concerned with surgery, but with operations and their associated pain. In the nineteenth century, the discovery of antisepsis countered the risk of infection, and the discovery of anaesthesia removed the pain. Yet, before these discoveries, painful, risky, and uncertain operations, while never desired or popular, were nonetheless an accepted form of treatment. Viewed from the experience of the twenty-first century, this acceptance is not easy to understand, but is in part explained by Pierre Dionis, who taught in the Royal Gardens in Paris under the patronage of King Louis XIV. He wrote:

> *When a Chirurgeon has without hesitation acquainted the Patient that he must of necessity resolve to die, or undergo the Operation, there are none but will choose the Operation. We are not willing to die; and tho' we are certain of suffering great Pains, we always prefer them to Death (2).*

This is not the only answer. The historical material cannot simply be viewed through the prism of modern concepts, knowledge, and behaviour. One writer wrote of history that it was '*An account, mostly false, of events, mostly unimportant, which are brought about by rulers, mostly knaves, and soldiers, mostly fools*' (3). This may be an exaggeration, but it points to the problem. A more elegant expression of the problem is: '*The past is a foreign country; they do things differently there*' (4).

The reality is that reactions to pain were different in the past. Before the late nineteenth century, there were no pain-killing medicaments except opium, which had serious side effects and was unpleasant to consume. There were medicines available from plants, but none of them were what we would call reliable or consistent. For the greatest part of human existence, pain was something that had to be endured, like it or not. Thus, people's reactions to it were different from reactions in the modern world. This needs to be understood.

This book examines what surgeons of earlier times had to say about the pain of an operation. Every attempt is made to place their remarks in the context of their own time. While the result is necessarily patchy and incomplete, it nonetheless permits the reader to examine development of a logical evolution of experience and attitudes. Where possible, details of each surgeon's background are included, since these affect the surgeon's personality, which in turn will impact his relationship with patients.

One final note. There are multiple quotations in the text. The reason is simple. It is proposed that repeating what people actually said is more reliable than presenting an interpretation of what was said. These quotations were either originally in English or have been taken from published English translations of other languages. English vocabulary, spelling, grammar, and syntax have changed over the centuries. The quotations have not been edited to conform to contemporary practice. Not even the punctuation has been changed.

Jeremy Ganz

REFERENCES

1. Bell J. *Preliminary Discourse on the Education and Duties of the Surgeon. The Principles of Surgery. I.* London: Thomas Tegg; 1826, pp. 1–14.
2. Dionis P. Of the Bubonocele. In *A Course of Cirurgical Operations*. London: Jacob Tonson; 1710, pp. 188–96.
3. Bierce A. *The Cynic's Word Book.* New York: Doubleday, Page & Company; 1906.
4. Hartley LP. *The Go-Between.* London: Hamish Hamilton; 1953.

Acknowledgements

Many years ago, while preparing for a PhD, I became fascinated by the practice of surgery in the past. Since retirement, it has become possible to pursue that interest. I have received advice and assistance from Cambridge University Emeritus Professor Sir Geoffrey Lloyd. Professor Vivian Nutton has also proffered frequent, prompt, and excellent advice. It was he who suggested that I should seek further information from Professor Michael McVaugh, whose book on medieval surgeons has been most valuable.

One of the difficulties in examining the history of surgery is the language barrier. It is thus that I offer profound thanks to the late Leonard D. Rosenman, who, in his retirement, translated the writings of the most influential medieval surgeons. Without his work, my studies would not have been possible. In addition, it is with great pleasure that I thank a fellow neurosurgeon-turned-translator, Ian Johnston. We have discussed the terminology of an instrument described in his translation of Galen's Method of Medicine Book VI, in the Loeb Classical Library series. His advice was invaluable.

I should also like to convey my thanks to the internet and the facilities that it provides, not least, access to ancient documents retained within the confines of distinguished libraries. Accessing such institutions involves the acquisition of permission to access their contents together with expenses of travel and accommodation while using the access so obtained. This still remains occasionally necessary, and I am grateful to the British Library, the Wellcome Library, and the Bodleian Library for their unstinting help.

Finally, like any author, I should like to thank my patient wife, Gao Nan Ping. Without her constant help and support, this book could not have been written.

Author Biography

Jeremy C. Ganz studied at the University of Cambridge, qualifying as a doctor in 1967 and obtaining the FRCS in 1973. His neurosurgical training was at the National Hospital for Nervous Diseases, Queen Square London; Frenchay Hospital, Bristol; and the Manchester Royal Infirmary. In 1976, he emigrated to Norway, and in 1978 acquired a Norwegian Medical License and the qualification of Specialist in Neurosurgery. He has practiced in Trondheim and Bergen. He was awarded a Doctor of Medicine degree by the University of Bergen in 1990. From 1993 to 2001, he taught the Gamma Knife technique in over seventy centres around the world, followed by six years in Cairo helping to establish the Gamma Knife Center there. In 2006, he returned to practice neurosurgery in Bergen, retiring in 2010. Thereafter, he spent a year teaching neurology in English at Shantou Medical University, Guandong Province, People's Republic of China. Since retirement in 2010, he has published four books on neurosurgery- and radiosurgery-related topics, and four books on the history of surgery.

Glossary

Word	Explanation	Chapters
	Anatomical	
Alveolar bone	The specialized bone in the jaw that forms the sockets (alveoli) which hold the roots of the teeth	7
Alveoli	Alveoli are tiny air sacs in the lungs where O_2 and CO_2 pass inwards and outwards.	4
Cerebellum	Little brain. The part of the brain at the back below the cerebrum	1
Cerebral	Concerning the cerebrum, the largest and most prominent part of the brain	1, 9
Clavicle	Collar bone	4
Coccyx	Tailbone. The lowest portion of the spine consisting of five vertebrae rigidly attached to each other	4
Collagen	The fibrous protein which is the major component of all connective tissue	2
Cooper's Pelvic Ligament	Thickening of the periosteum along the upper surface of the pubic bone	11
Cooper's Ligament of Breast	Network of fibrous connective tissue in the breast. Provides support, and attaches skin to the chest wall	11
Cornea	Transparent part of the wall of the eye through which light passes	8
Cranium	Another word for the skull	6, 7, 9, 10
Diarrhoea	Loose watery stools	4, 7, 10, 11
Distal	Situated away from the centre of the body or from the point of attachment	10, 11
Dura	The outer membrane around the brain, adherent to the skull's interior, forms folds between brain parts	7, 10
Elastin	A key structural protein in the connective tissue which provides elasticity	2
Epithelium	Layer of cells covering body surfaces in contact with the exterior. Skin and mucosa	4, 11
Fetus	The developing embryo from around the ninth week. This is the correct spelling as it is a Latin word.	4
Foramen	Opening	10
Humerus	The bone of the upper arm	3
Iliac Spine	The part of the bony pelvis which can be felt low down at the sides of the abdomen	8
Inguinal	Relating to the groin	4, 7, 9, 11
Jugular Veins	Major veins in the neck which drain blood from the brain and cranium	4
Lateral Ventricles	Two of the central fluid filled spaces within the brain	13
Lumbar Region	Lower part of the back and spine just above the pelvis	4
Lumen	The lumen is the space within the walls of a tube	2

(*Continued*)

Word	Explanation	Chapters
Lymph Nodes	Collections of cells in the lymphatic system which filter the lymph and immune cells which attack foreign cells	7
Lymphatic System	A separate system of vessels which drain excess fluids from the tissues and return them to the blood	7
Mucous Membrane	The moist layer of cells covering the gastrointestinal, respiratory, and urogenital systems.	7
Occiput	The backmost portion of the cranium	4
Pericranium	The membrane which covers and nourishes the exterior surface of the bones of the skull	6
Perineum/Perineal	The region between the anus and the genitals	12
Proximal	Situated closer to the centre of the body or the point of attachment.	7, 11
Sciatic Nerve	Longest nerve. Runs from the back through the buttocks to the back of the leg to the foot	13, 14
Third Ventricle	One of the central fluid-filled spaces within the brain into which the lateral ventricles drain.	10
Tonsils	Two clumps of lymphoid tissue at the back of the throat	7, 8, 9
Trachea	The part of the respiratory system connecting the larynx to the bronchi	7
Transversalis Fascia	Layer of tissue lining the inner abdominal wall, between the transversus abdominis muscle and peritoneum	11
Umbilicus	Navel	4, 8
Urethra	The portion of the urogenital system between the bladder and the exterior	3, 11, 12
Urogenital	Related to the urinary and reproductive systems	11
Vertebra	A component bone of the spinal column	3, 4
	Biographical	
Avicenna	Avicenna (ca. 980–1037), a most important physician whose medical texts were influential for centuries	4, 5
Rhazes	Rhazes (c.865–925), an important Persian physician	4
	Humoural	
Phlegmatic	Behaviour associated with the humour 'Phlegm'. See chapter 2	2, 4
Phlegmons	Diffuse areas of inflammation	9
	Pathological	
Abscess	A pocket of pus formed in the body	1, 3, 4, 5, 7, 8, 9, 11, 12, 14
Anal/Perianal Fistula	A tunnel that forms between the anal canal and the skin near the anus	3, 6, 8, 9, 11
Apoplexy	A sudden loss of consciousness accompanied by paralysis	4
Ataxia	Unsteady gait. Comes from a Greek word. ἀ (a) = without Τάξις (taxia) = arrangement	1
Bacteria	Single-celled organisms without a nucleus. They invade the body, multiply, and do damage.	2, 7
Bone Caries	The progressive destruction and decay of bone	8, 9, 10

(*Continued*)

Word	Explanation	Chapters
Cancer	A tumour which spreads locally by invasion and at a distance by parts spreading in blood and lymph	3, 4, 7, 8, 9, 11
Carbuncles	A cluster of interconnected abscesses	3, 7
Carcinoma	A cancer arising from an epithelium (see above)	11
Contusion	A painful swelling due to blood leaking into the tissues following blunt trauma damaging blood vessels	4, 6, 9, 11
Dactylitis	An inflammation of a digit	7
Denaturation	Destruction of the structure of a protein with loss of function, since function relies on shape	2
Dyspnoea	Shortness of breath	4
Ectropion	A condition where a weakened lower eyelid drooped outwards failing to cover the eye	3
Emboli	A detached mass, within a blood vessel, clot, fat, or air which may be carried elsewhere to block vessels	10
Entropion	Inverted eyelids resulting in eyelashes scratching the eye	3, 7
Epilepsy	Recurrent, unprovoked seizures	3, 4, 6, 7
Eschar	A piece of dead tissue that has become hard and dry. Often dark and crusty. Commonest after burns.	2, 3, 7
Fistula	An abnormal connection between two epithelial surfaces (See above)	3, 4, 6, 7, 8, 9, 10, 11
Gangrene	Death of parts of the body deprived of a blood supply	2, 3, 4, 6, 7, 8, 9, 11
Granulation Tissue	Tissue formed from new blood vessels that brings nutrients, oxygen, and cells to the grainy looking healing tissue	2, 7, 11
Granulations	See granulation tissue	12
Gumma	A persistent local region of granulation tissue with central necrosis appearing in the late stages of syphilis	7
Haemorrhoids	Swollen and inflamed veins in the anus or lower rectum, also known as piles	3, 4, 7, 8, 9, 12
Hare Lip	A defect in the upper lip due to faulty development and showing as a cleft in the lip	8
Hernia	A weakness in the wall of a body cavity permitting contents to displace external to that cavity	3, 4, 7, 8, 9, 11
Hydatid Cyst	A parasitic infection caused by a tapeworm	11
Hydrocele	An accumulation of a clear, yellow, watery (serous) fluid in a body cavity	3, 4, 7, 8, 9, 11
Hypospadias	A condition where the opening of the urethra is under the penis and further back than the tip	3
Incarcerated Hernia	A hernia, the contents of which cannot be replaced to their normal situation	8
Inflammation	Physical reaction to injury or infection with warmth, redness, pain, and swelling	1, 3, 7, 8, 9, 11, 12
Inguinal Hernia	A swelling in the groin due to a weakness of the adjacent abdominal wall	4, 7, 11
Ischaemia	The changes following inadequate blood supply to a tissue	10
Issues	Little ulcers made by surgeons in various parts of the body and kept open by patients	2, 7

(*Continued*)

Word	Explanation	Chapters
Lachrymal Fistula	Abnormal passage which directs the tears to the skin	4, 7, 8
Nasal Polyp	Soft benign growth in the lining of the nose and paranasal sinuses	7, 8, 9, 10, 11
Necrosis	Death of cells	2, 7
Oedema	An abnormal accumulation of water in the tissues between the cells	2
Ophthalmia	An inflammation of the eye and especially the conjunctiva	3
Osteitis	Bone inflammation	8
Paronychia	An inflammation located where the skin meets the side of a nail. It is excruciating	7, 11, 14
Phimosis	Foreskin too tight to be pulled back over the head of the penis	9
Pleurisy	Inflammation of the pleura which is the membrane surrounding the lungs and lining the thorax,	4
Ranula	A fluid-filled cyst which forms in the mouth usually under the tongue	7
Scrofula	Infection of neck lymph nodes by tuberculosis	4, 7
Scrofulous	Tuberculous	10
Spina Ventosa	Outdated term for cystic enlargement of bones due to tuberculosis	9
Steatoma	A synonym for a sebaceous cyst	8
Suppuration	Formation and discharge of pus	2, 8, 9, 10, 11, 12
Syphilis	A sexually transmitted infection	7
Tenesmus	The feeling of passing a stool when the bowel is empty	8
Thrombosis	Blood clot within the confines of a blood vessel	10
Tuberculosis	A disease caused by a bacterium. It mainly affects lungs but may affect any organ including lymph nodes	7, 9
Ulcer	A region where the surface epithelium is missing revealing diseased underlying tissue	2, 4, 7, 8, 9, 10, 11
Ulcer, Callous	Chronic non-healing ulcers with a hard base and inelastic margins	7
Ulcer, Vitiated	An ulcer where the appearances of the matter is green acrid and gelatinous, differing from pus	9
Varices	Swollen enlarged veins	3
Varicocele	A swelling of the veins of the scrotum	12
Venereal	Relating to sexual intercourse, desire, or disease	9
Vitiligo	A long-term skin condition where patches of skin lose their colour	3
	Therapeutic	
Amputation	Removal of part of a limb	2, 3, 4, 7, 8, 9, 10, 11, 13, 14
Apposed	Brought together	2, 6,
Caesarean Section	Opening the womb through an abdominal incision to deliver a baby	7, 9
Counterirritation	Making a pain in one location to diminish pain in another	2, 3, 4, 6, 7

(Continued)

Word	Explanation	Chapters
Haemorrhoidectomy	The excision of haemorrhoids	3, 4, 11
Haemostasis	Stopping haemorrhage	2, 4, 7, 8, 10, 13
Lithotomy	The removal of bladder stones. Usually involving an incision from below in front of the anus	2, 3, 4, 7, 8, 10, 11, 12, 14
Lithotrity	Crushing bladder stones within the bladder	12
Mastectomy	Removal of a breast	9, 12, 14
Orchiectomy	Removal of a testis	9
Paracentesis (abdominal)	A procedure to remove fluid from the abdomen	8
Phlebotomy	An opening in a blood vessel to let out blood and thereby balance the humours in the body (see page)	3, 4, 6, 7, 8, 9, 10, 11, 12
Proximal Artery Ligation	Ligate the femoral artery inches above an aneurysm behind the knee. Collateral circulation supplies blood.	11
Seton	A surgical thread or strip of material inserted under the skin to facilitate drainage or keep a wound open	6, 7, 11
Speculum	A medical tool for investigating body orifices	7
Tincture	A solution in alcohol	7, 11
Tonsillectomy	Excision of the tonsils	4, 8, 9, 11, 12
Tracheostomy	An opening in the trachea below the larynx which permits respiration when the upper airway is blocked	3
Tracheotomy	Making an opening in the trachea to permit passage of air when the upper airways are blocked	7, 9
Trepanation	Trepanation is the procedure of removing pieces of cranium to gain access to the interior	4, 6, 7, 8, 10
Trocar	A hollow instrument with a sharp tip which can gain access to a body cavity	8
Venepuncture	An opening in a vein to let out blood and thereby balance the humours in the body (see phlebotomy)	3, 7
Venesection	See phlebotomy	12

1 Some Aspects of Pain Including the Pains of Surgery

DEFINITIONS

It is impossible to define what has not been created by the definer, and this applies to pain. Definitions of pain are really descriptions. It is comforting in the twenty-first century to have a respected institution tell us what things mean. In 1974, the International Association for the Study of Pain (IASP) was formed, and it is the accepted authority. Its 'definition' is, in principle, accurate but lacks impact. It informs us that pain is: '*An unpleasant sensory and emotional experience associated with, or resembling that associated with, actual or potential tissue damage*'. A description that seems to encompass more of the reality of the experience of pain was written by an American physician called Victor Robinson, who died in 1947. He wrote: '*Pain is the cruel but life-saving guardian of protoplasm*' [1].

Before proceeding, it is necessary to specify what this book is not about. Books on the history of pain cover a number of topics. These include 'definitions' of the nature of pain, the interrelation between the sufferer and the culture and environment, and the body processes underlying the experienced pain [2–5]. We all understand what we mean by pain, even if we cannot understand how it works. However, while definitions or descriptions may be useful for research workers, it is difficult to believe that familiarity with them will relieve the suffering of a fractured collarbone. Understanding the nature of pain is not what a sufferer requires. Such an unfortunate individual needs only one thing; the application of a treatment which will make the pain go away. That is the topic of this book.

COMBATTING PAIN

Since pain is unpleasant, it has always been natural to seek ways of stopping it. From the early days, it has been known that the consumption of substances may help. This seems to be a non-conscious property since non-human animals are known to seek certain plants that may soothe pain. This is called zoopharmacognosy, and it is widespread. Using plants for self-medication has been noted in elephants, bison, wild boar, pigs, tigers, dogs, bears, jackals, wolves, rhinoceroses, and monkeys [6]. Thus, using plants for self-medication does not necessarily require the self-awareness specific to humankind [7]. Where humanity differs is in the development of chemicals that have more profound effects than native plants. Of these chemicals, alcohol [8] and opium [9] are the most well-known, and they were synthesized and used either for pleasure or to combat pain before the invention of writing. Nonetheless, Alcohol

DOI: 10.1201/9781003748816-1

and opium were not the only substances used to improve upon the medicines provided by nature. There are a number of preparations mentioned in classical literature. Thus, Homer described 'Nepenthe' and also 'Helenium' made from the tears of Helen of Troy. These are mythical and their nature is not known. Nonetheless, there were real agents. There were also Hellebore, Mandragora, Hemlock, Henbane, and even Lettuce [1]. The accessibility, cost, and reputation of these preparations are of course, not known.

UNDERSTANDING PAIN

There is another way in which we humans differ in our response to pain, and that certainly is a consequence of our advanced cerebral activity. One feature of that activity is curiosity, and its importance has been noted by the greatest thinkers. Aristotle wrote:

> *All men by nature are actuated with the desire of knowledge [10].*

Over two millennia later, Albert Einstein wrote:

> *The important thing is not to stop questioning. Curiosity has its own reason for existence [11].*

Curiosity drives us to explain whatever matters to us, and there is a multitude of phenomena requiring explanation. One method of supplying such explanations in primitive societies was to invent supernatural explanations. These included imagined deities usually administered by priesthoods. This was reasonable in societies that lacked the technology to examine and analyse natural phenomena. The priests of Ancient Egypt [12] and the Asklepiads of Ancient Greece [13] are examples of this.

With Hippocrates' documentation of illnesses and their treatment came a new rational approach to medicine. He outlined a system of humoral pathology that would influence medical thinking for two millennia. It is considered in more detail in later chapters. However, the crucial point is that these concepts represented a non-supernatural explanation of the causes of pain, even if it was in fact nonsense. As time passed, European history discouraged curiosity, preferring the safety of accepted opinion. There would be little significant intellectual effort to improve the understanding of the treatment of pain until the Renaissance.

ABSENCE OF EFFECTIVE ANALGESIA

How we react is much affected by what we can expect. In the modern world, relatively minor pain from such causes as headache, toothache, and earache may be relieved by tablets that can be bought at pharmacies over the counter without a prescription. More severe pains will require a prescription. Up to the nineteenth century, no reliable painkillers existed, with the emphasis on reliable. In the early part of that century, codeine became obtainable, although it has the disadvantages of addiction and sedation. It can also induce constipation. The origin of the name is not obvious, but like opium, the substance comes from the head of the opium poppy. The name 'codeine' comes from a Greek word (κοδέια), which means poppy head. At the end of the 1890s, aspirin came on the market. In the modern world, pain relief in one form or another is widely available and hence expected.

On the other hand, for most of history there were no available reliable analgesics. This lack must have influenced people's expectations. Unsurprisingly, this lack is not documented because commenting on the lack of something that is unknown is impossible. With this general experience, it would seem likely that since pain could not be avoided, many sufferers would accept that they had no choice but to grin and bear the pain.

COMPLEXITY OF REACTIONS TO PAIN

Even in modern times, with readily accessible painkillers, there are a variety of situations where pain is better tolerated. The first such situation is the battlefield.

Battlefield Injuries

There is a study from the Second World War on 215 men, wounded while fighting in Italy. There were five groups of injuries. These were compound fractures[1] of long bones, extensive soft tissue wounds, penetrating wounds of the thorax, penetrating wounds of the abdomen, and penetrating wounds of the brain. The patients were asked whether they wanted pain relief medication, shortly after admission to the hospital. Only 27% requested it. It was also noted that patients in shock were more distressed by thirst than by pain. Beecher speculated on the low need for analgesia in these patients, but did not provide further data to clarify the nonetheless solid findings [14].

The German surgeon Ferdinand Sauerbruch commented on the experience of Napoleon's field physician Dominique Jean Larrey. Sauerbruch wrote:

> *a remarkable feature of his accounts, which describe the nature and severity of the wounds in great detail, is how rarely they refer directly to pain. His men accepted pain as a matter of course, and he knew that he could alleviate it psychologically. In this respect it is interesting to note that his attitude to the problem was quite different from ours today: there was no need to talk much about pain; it was something which was present in any case and was therefore accepted as natural [15].*

In 1965, Melzack and Wall introduced new theories about the mechanisms underlying the experience of pain. In due course, Wall wrote a book about the science of pain, which includes references to the lack of correlation between injury and pain. He starts with a picture from the Battle of Khandaq at Medina (see Figure 1.1). The picture shows the leaders of the two sides. Imam Ali (on the left), the cousin and son-in-law of Mohamed has just cut off the left leg of Amr Bin Wid (on the right), who was the leader of the forces laying siege to Medina. Bin Wid is holding his leg in his hand prior to throwing it at Ali, who then killed him. This is taken to indicate that Bin Wid was unaffected by the pain he could have been expected to experience. Wall continues by presenting evidence from the Yom Kippur War, where injured soldiers seldom complained of pain [16].

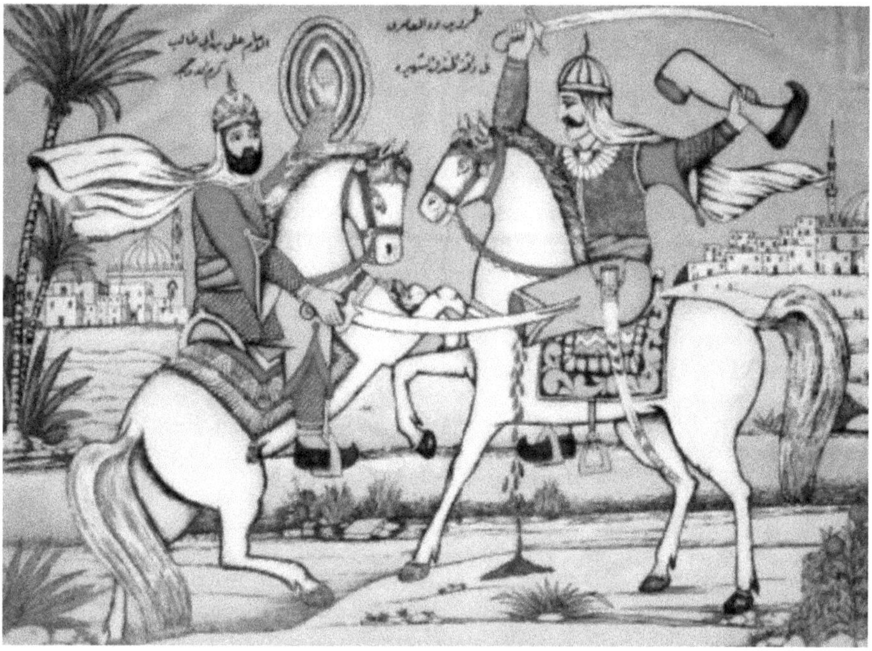

FIGURE 1.1 Scene from the battle of Khandaq at Medina.

Fight between Imam Ali and Amr Bin Wid (see text).

Sport and Pain

Toleration of pain is not restricted to the stress of the battlefield. There are individuals who go to great lengths to acquire expertise for a sport where injury is either a part of the sport itself, for example, boxing, or where it is an unwanted but unavoidable consequence of risks taken during the sport, as in horseracing. Dick Francis, in his autobiography 'The Sport of Queens' wrote:

> *The ability of his body to absorb and disregard bangs and breaks is one of the things which make it possible for a man to be a steeplechase jockey, and because of his hard fitness the effect his injuries have on him should not be judged by the effect they would have on an average man. Jockeys feel the same pain but it passes sooner, and except when the injury is serious and complicated they heal faster [17].*

Pain and Courage

In many societies, a painful initiation from adolescent to adult has been a necessary trial for young men. Such rituals established that the individual had the ability to cope with pain, an ability that would be an important component of that individual's self-respect and would be a source of admiration by those aware of it. It may be discovered in all sorts of situations. Perhaps the most limited is the pain associated with training and performing contact sports. Those who enter a burning building to save a child or an old person are even more admired. The young men who lost their lives or who were injured on the beaches of northern France on D-Day 1944 are among those we most admire. A corollary of this acquired admiration is the knowledge for any individual that behaving in this way will improve his/her standing and increase his/her self-respect.

While courage during sport, hunting, or war is well recognized, tales of such courage endured during the course of surgery are not common, but there are two well-known examples. One from Ancient Rome concerns a general. The story was related by Plutarch in his biography of the Roman general and seven times consul, Gaius Marius (157 to 86 BC).

> *Both his legs, it is said, had become varicose, and as he disliked this deformity, he resolved to put himself in the surgeon's hands. Accordingly he presented to the surgeon one of his legs without allowing himself to be bound; and without making a single movement or uttering a single groan, with steady countenance and in silence he endured excessive pain during the operation. But when the surgeon was going to take the other leg, Marius refused to present it, saying that he perceived the cure was not worth the pain [18].*

The second account of great bravery does not concern a mature adult like Marius but a sixteen-year-old boy, who would later become Henry V of England. He was struck on the left side of his face [19] by an arrow from a longbow [20]. The arrow buried itself to a depth of 6 inches, but fortunately it did not injure any life-dependent structures. Henry refused to leave the field of the battle, which his father, Henry IV, eventually won [21]. The shaft of the arrow was pulled out, probably by Henry himself, leaving the arrowhead in situ at a depth of 6 inches. Afterwards, he was seen by a number of surgeons who proposed potions and other unsuccessful cures, which delayed effective treatment for presumably a few days. He was then seen by a surgeon called John Bradmore. This gentleman introduced what he called tents into the wound. These were made by wrapping linen around elder pith. This is the soft, spongy core of dead elder branches. These cylinders were introduced down to the retained arrowhead. Using broader and broader cylinders, the track of the arrow was dilated until Bradmore could introduce an instrument of his own design made for the purpose during the treatment. This attached itself to the arrowhead, which was withdrawn [19]. This injury, with the subsequent treatment spread over many days, must have been agony for the teenage victim, but clearly, he tolerated it to go on to gain the crown and fight the Battle of Agincourt.

Pain and Christianity

The importance of the soul exceeding the importance of the body is an important component of Christian belief. How this applies to pain is neatly encompassed within the Ancrene Riwle, a medieval code of rules for the life of women living in reclusion, written specifically for three sisters who had retired to a life of prayer and penance but not within an institution.

> *Now the remedy against sickness visited by God is fortitude: be patient, and thank God for his favour in selecting and testing you in this way. And as regards ill-health caused by immoderation or folly, beg his mercy and forgiveness because you have through your own stupidity so damaged your body that you may no longer serve him as you ought... Thus sickness brings spiritual healing, and cures the wounds of the soul, and prevents it from sustaining further damage, as it surely would had God not intervened [22].*

These accepted teachings placed additional pressure on the individual who was required to tolerate pain as evidence of God's goodwill or as a punishment for not living up to God's requirements.

CLINICAL PATTERNS OF PAIN

The body receives conscious information via five senses: vision, hearing, smell, taste, and touch. While not a sense, pain is a sensation and shares with the senses physical and mental components with a great deal of variability. There is, however, one difference from the senses. While all the senses can, in excess, produce sensations that are unpleasant, pain alone is unpleasant by definition. The clinical pattern of pains is, for convenience, divided into acute and chronic. Chronic pain is the topic of much modern writing but is not relevant in the current context, since its duration far exceeds that of any surgical operation [2–4]. Acute pain is caused by illness or injury. Examples of pain caused by illness are toothache, appendicitis, or renal colic. These pains start quickly and persist for several hours or a day or two. They persist until either their cause resolves spontaneously or until therapy is successful. Unlike the pain of an operation, their course and intensity are unpredictable.

CHARACTERISTICS OF SURGICAL PAIN

A surgical operation prior to the availability of anaesthesia was a painful experience with uncertain benefit. Why did people allow themselves to undergo it? The simple answer was the belief that the pain of surgery was less than the pain that would develop in the absence of treatment. This means a consideration of causes and effects. For most of recorded history, the ability to examine the relationship between cause and effect existed only for events and experiences that were immediately available to the senses. Being wounded was one such experience. From earliest times, wound treatment required some means of bringing the edges together and keeping them in apposition. Failure to do so would result in infection. There was no understanding of the nature of the infection, but one aspect of such sepsis would have been most obvious to the sufferer. Contaminated wounds stink. In ancient Sumer, war was a constant background to the developing society [23]. The same is true of ancient Egypt [24]. It was also true in ancient Greece [25], and the Roman Empire was based on the activities of its powerful army [26]. Thus, in those far-off times, the pain of wounds and the pain of their treatment management would have been familiar.

The pain of an operation would last a maximum of two hours, and in most cases for a much shorter period. Its course and intensity would be largely predictable, being determined at the discretion of the operating surgeon. While its intention was therapeutic, its cause was an injury. Familiar causes of injuries are accidents, crime, or military action, though these differ from the pain of surgery. In most injuries, there are two kinds of pain. There is pain produced by the inflicting agent, which is brief, lasting a few seconds. This is followed by pain arising from tissue damaged as a result of the injury and is of variable intensity. By contrast, the pain inflicted during surgery could persist for minutes or even hours. It has no parallel in other activities, except perhaps torture.

THE PATIENT SURGEON RELATIONSHIP

There are many tales of the arrogance and brutality of surgeons [2–4, 27]. There is a widespread belief that those who undergo a medical education and surgical training suffer an inescapable dehumanizing effect from these experiences. It is inescapable that since surgeons are human and varied, regrettably, some will behave badly. On the other hand, my experience is that surgeons learn to cope with the harsher aspects of their work, but they do not become unaware of them. Without an anaesthetic, patients suffer the worst agony, but they only suffer it once. The surgeon experiences patients' expressions of distress repeatedly over a career lasting many years. Inevitably, surgical training accustoms students to tolerate the uncomfortable sides of their profession to be.

All too little has been written about the relationship from the surgeon's point of view. The interaction between surgeon and patient is inevitably uneven. The patient has a need, and the surgeon can hopefully provide for that need. This unevenness can be difficult for the patient, and the attitudes and activities of surgeons are examined with a view to attaching criticism. This is well expressed by that icon of quality, humanity, and surgery, Ambroise Paré, surgeon to four kings of France and a man who revolutionized wound treatment by stopping the universal use of cautery after gunshot wounds. He wrote:

> *A Chirurgeon must have a strong, stable, and intrepid hand, and a mind resolute and merciless; so that to heal him he taketh in hand, he be not moved to make more haste than the thing requires; or to cut less than is needfull; but which doeth all things as if he were nothing affected with their cries; not giving heed to the judgement of the vain common people, who speak ill of Chirurgeons because of their ignorance [28].*

The barrier between the surgeon and the public was clearly expressed by a surgeon called J. Chalmers Da Costa (1863 to 1933) who wrote:

> *A test as to whether or not a practitioner of medicine has or has not the spirit of the quack is the direction to which he looks for reputation. The decent man seeks reputation among the members of his own profession; the other sort of person attempts to gain notoriety with the general public. As Sir James Paget said, such notoriety may be obtained by the most ignorant "through self-assertion, self -advertising, or mere impudence." [29]*

REGULATION OF SURGEONS

Despite all the difficulties the practice of surgery entails, and the criticisms that surgeons often experience as unjust, there remains one indisputable fact. Patients have required surgeons at least since the time of Hammurabi (2250 BC). We know this with certainty because Hammurabi was responsible for a list of regulations governing surgical practice. The regulations included 215 to 223.

> *§ 215*
> *If a physician operate on a man for a severe wound (or make a severe wound upon a man) with a bronze lancet and save the man's life; or if he open an abscess (in the eye) of a man with a bronze lancet and save that man's eye, he shall receive ten shekels of silver (as his fee).*
>
> *§ 216*
> *If he be a freeman, he shall receive five shekels.*
>
> *§ 217*
> *If it be a man's slave, the owner of the slave shall give two shekels of silver to the physician.*
>
> *§ 218*
> *If a physician operate on a man for a severe wound with a bronze lancet and cause that man's death; or open an abscess (in the eye) of a man with a bronze lancet and destroy the man's eye, they shall cut off his fingers.*
>
> *§ 219*
> *If a physician operate on a slave of a freeman for a severe wound with a bronze lancet and cause his death, he shall restore a slave of equal value.*
>
> *§ 220*
> *If he open an abscess (in his eye) with a bronze lancet, and destroy his eye, he shall pay silver to extent of one-half of his price.*
>
> *§ 221*
> *If a physician set a broken bone for a man or cure his diseased bowels, the patient shall give five shekels of silver to the physician.*
>
> *§ 222*
> *If he be a freeman, he shall give three shekels of silver.*
>
> *§ 223*
> *If it be a man's slave, the owner of the slave shall give two shekels of silver to the physician.*

Five shekels was equivalent to the yearly rent of a good type of house and represented 150 times the daily wage of a workman. However, Hammurabi´s Code might have discouraged the pursuit of a career in Ophthalmology given the severity of the penalties for surgical misadventure. It is noteworthy that the penalties were related to the socioeconomic status of the patient. So, at this early date, surgical practice was to be guided by the law of the land, and the guidance was stringent [30]. The surgeon may have been well paid, but few, if any, subsequent regulations of practice have included such draconian punishments.

CONTEMPORARY PAINFUL TREATMENT WITHOUT ANAESTHESIA

It might be thought that modern surgeons have no idea about painful treatment without the benefit of relief. This is not so. There are still painful treatments performed without anaesthesia. These include reduction of the dislocation of the shoulder or the jaw. This is most easily done with a sitting patient and as soon as possible after the injury, since delay is accompanied by swelling of the surrounding tissues, making reduction more difficult. The responsible surgeon knows that the procedure will hurt the patient, but he/she knows that reduction is usually simple and that it will lead to an immediate, dramatic reduction in the pain. Knowing this, the pain of reduction feels an acceptable price to pay for almost instant relief. Usually, the sudden relief from pain following reduction induces an incomparable gratitude in the patient.

UNAVOIDABLE LIMITATIONS

One of the difficulties in studying surgical history and writing about it is the number of skills required to obtain a balanced picture. For example, historians are specially trained to be able to read original documents in foreign and often ancient languages. They also have superior skills in relating texts to what is known of the author and how that author relates to others. These are skills beyond the capability of most surgeons. On the other hand, the historian lacks the experience of a lifetime of dealing with sick people, and their reactions to surgery and surgeons. This author is, or rather was, a surgeon and has a lifetime of managing the results of disease. For example, with experience, diagnoses can on occasion be made by simply looking at a patient. There is a condition called ataxia (this comes from a Greek word ἀ (a) = without Τάξις (taxia) = arrangement). It is a condition of unsteady gait. It can arise from diseases in two locations, the cerebellum (little brain) at the back of the head and the spinal cord. Cerebellar ataxia arises from a failure of the brain's computer to organize the nervous impulses required to produce coordinated movement. The patient looks ahead. Spinal ataxia comes from a lesion in the spinal cord, preventing the brain from knowing where the legs are. In consequence, the patient looks downwards at the ground.

CONCLUSIONS

Pain is a complex, unpleasant sensory experience. Its intensity and tolerability vary between individuals and circumstances. Chapter 2 examines the relationship between pain and specific procedures. It also considers a most agonizing but historically popular treatment called cauterization, which involved burning the body to treat diseases. Thereafter, the rest of this book examines how surgeons and patients managed the unavoidable rigours of an operation while wide awake and unanaesthetized.

As this chapter indicates, many influences form the background to the experience of a surgical operation. The following chapters will describe how these influences worked in practice.

NOTE

1 Compound fractures are fractures accompanied by wounds so that the injured bone is exposed to the external milieu.

REFERENCES

1. Robinson V. *Early Developments. Victory over Pain.* New York: Henry Schuman; 1946, pp. 3–44.
2. Bourke J. *The Story of Pain.* Oxford: Oxford University Press; 2014.
3. Wall P. *Pain: The Science of Suffering.* London: Weidenfeld and Nicolson; 2000.
4. Morris DB. *The Culture of Pain.* Berkeley, CA: University of California Press; 1991.
5. Rey R. *The History of Pain.* Cambridge, MA: Harvard University Press; 1993.
6. Huffman MA. Animal Self-Medication and Ethno-Medicine: Exploration and Exploitation of the Medicinal Properties of Plants. *Proceedings of the Nutrition Society.* 2003; 62: 371–381.
7. Engel C. *Wild Health: How Animals Keep Themselves Well and What We Can Learn From Them.* Hawthorne, CA: GF Books; 2021.
8. McGovern PE. *Uncorking the Past.* Berkeley, CA: University of California Press; 2010.
9. Salavert A, Zazzo A, Martin L, Antolín F, Gauthier C, Thil F, et al. Direct Dating Reveals the Early History of Opium Poppy in Western Europe. *Scientific Reports.* 2020; 10.
10. Aristotle. *Metaphysics.* London: Henry G. Bohn; 1857.
11. Einstein A. Old Man's Advice to Youth: 'Never Lose a Holy Curiosity'. *Life.* 1955; 2: 64.
12. Allen JP. *The Art of Medicine in Ancient Egypt. The Art of Medicine in Ancient Egypt.* New Haven, CT: Yale University Press; 2005, pp. 9–14.
13. Guthrie D. *Early Greek Medicine. A History of Medicine.* London: Thomas Nelson and Sons Ltd; 1960, pp. 39–50.
14. Beecher HK. Pain. *Surgical Clinics of North America.* 1963; 43: 609–618.
15. Roby C. *Galen on Pain.* Ann Arbor, MI: Columbia; 2005.
16. Wall P. *Private Pain and Public Display. Pain: The Science of Suffering.* London: Weidenfeld and Nicolson; 2000, pp. 1–14.
17. Francis D. *The Sport of Queens.* London: Penguin Books; 1988.
18. Plutarch. *Life of Gaius Marius. Plutarch's Lives Volume 2.* London: George Bell and Sons; 1899, pp. 221–284.
19. Lang SJ. *The "Philomena" of John Bradmore and its Middle English Derivative: A Perspective of Surgery in Late Medieval England.* St. Andrews: University of St. Andrews; 1998.
20. Jones D. *Henry V.* London: Head of Zeus; 2024.
21. Mortimer I. *1415. Henry V's Year of Glory.* London: Vintage 2010; 2009.
22. Rawcliffe C. *Diseases of the Soul. Medicine and Society in later Medieval England.* Stroud: Sutton Publishin; 1995, pp. 1–28.
23. Kramer SN. *The Sumerians.* Chicago, IL: The University of Cargo Press; 1963.
24. Breasted JH. *A History of Egypt.* New York: Charles Scribner's Sons; 1905.
25. Nomikos N. Injuries in the Greek Epics of Homer. *Chinese Journal of Traumatology.* 2018; 21: 109–112.

26. Britannica EoE. *Legion 2025*. Available from: https://www.britannica.com/topic/legion
27. Wear A. *Surgery: The Handwork of Medicine. Knowledge & Practice in English Medicine, 1550 - 1680*. Cambridge, MA: Cambridge University Press; 2004, pp. 210–274.
28. Johnson T. An Introduction or Compendious Way to Chirurgery: Of Chirurgical Operations. In *The Workes of the Famous Chirurgion Ambroise Pare: Translated out of the Latine and Compared with the French*. London: Richard Cotes; 1649, pp. 1–2.
29. DaCosta JC. *Certain Tendencies in Medicine. Selections from the Papers and Speeches of John Chalmers DaCosta*. Philadelphia, PA: W.B. Saunders Company; 1931, pp. 358–378.
30. Harper RF. *The Code of Hammurabi*. Chicago, IL: University of Chicago; 1904.

2 The Relationship between Surgical Procedures and Pain

INTRODUCTION

In this chapter, some of the commonest sources of pain during surgery prior to the introduction of anaesthesia will be considered.

PAIN INFLICTED BY HANDS OR INSTRUMENTS

Wound Treatment

In the regulations from Babylon in the Code of Hammurabi, the most common condition requiring an operation was a wound. The treatment of wounds has always been a major part of surgery. The principles governing this treatment have remained consistent down the ages. They were first properly documented in written texts during the times of ancient Greece.

The process passes through certain specific stages. Firstly, any significant haemorrhage from either arteries or veins must be stopped, a process called haemostasis from αἵματος or haemat meaning blood and στάσις or stasis meaning stopping. This will reduce the risk to life. It is also necessary because blood in the wound obscures the nature and severity of the damage. In most cases, pressure stops venous bleeding, but most life-threatening haemorrhage comes from arteries. These can also be closed with pressure, but this is not a reliable method. For smaller arteries, the vessel may be grasped and twisted in such a way that the lumen of the artery is closed and bleeding stops. (The lumen is the space within the walls of a vessel, which holds the blood.) For larger vessels, more dependable methods are required. The first of these involves passing a thread around the offending artery to make a loop and then tying the thread in such a way as to close the artery and stop the bleeding. This is called a ligature. The second method is to use heat. The heat must be intense enough to cause cellular water to vaporize and proteins to denature and coagulate. As proteins coagulate, the structural integrity of blood vessels is compromised, causing them to seal off and stop bleeding [1]. The modern equivalent of this technique is called diathermy, which uses electricity and is applied under anaesthesia. In Ancient Times, it was done using metal heated in a fire in a process called cautery, which was very painful and is considered below.

Another method to achieve haemostasis involved the use of chemicals called styptics. These worked in a variety of ways. Local blood vessels constricted, reducing blood flow. The tissues contracted, squeezing the blood vessels. Chemical properties caused blood to coagulate. Some styptics formed compounds with blood

 DOI: 10.1201/9781003748816-2

proteins, which physically closed damaged vessels. This was less painful initially than cautery, but styptics could not be applied with the same precision as cautery, and injury to surrounding tissues could not be avoided. Also, the end result of the process was a scar called an eschar, and this was not always strong enough to maintain the closure of the blood vessels [2].

The second stage of wound management is called wound toilet. This involves removing foreign material such as soil, sand, organic debris such as loose pieces of skin and bone fragments, and pieces of metal such as broken knife blades or bullets. It also enables the surgeon to determine the extent of a wound. It is another painful procedure. Ideally, all the foreign material should be removed because of the way the body resists infections. The body's defences are brought to a wound by the blood, where they can in different ways kill and remove the bacteria which cause infections. Since the non-living material has no blood supply, the defences cannot reach the attached bacteria, which are thus free to multiply. Even so, with the passage of time it was appreciated that finding and removing small fragments buried deep in a wound could result in more damage than the original injury, and such exhaustive searches became less popular [3].

The different tissues involved in wounds vary in their sensitivity to pain. The skin is a very pain-sensitive structure involved in all wounds. The membrane that covers bones is also markedly pain sensitive. As expected, injured nerves are very painful, and please note that partial injury is worse than total division. This will be discussed later in relation to bloodletting. With the poorer vision of surgery prior to the development of operating theatres and electric lights, the presence of nerves would not always have been easy to detect. Finally, it should not be forgotten that the instruments and other materials used by the surgeon could, by their design or by their application, contribute to the production of pain.

The final stage is wound closure, which involves one of two methods. If the wound edges are clean-cut and can easily be apposed, they should be kept apposed using sutures, plasters, or bandages. Sutures were another source of pain. In addition, the wound would experience tolerable soreness unless it became infected. If the edges were uneven, crushed, and there was associated tissue loss, no attempt should be made to sew the wound together. Instead, it should be allowed to heal from the bottom upwards, which involves the development of granulation tissue. (Granulation tissue is formed from new blood vessels, which bring oxygen and nutrients to the healing tissue. Blood clotting not only stops bleeding but also forms a matrix of blood proteins along which fibroblasts enter the region. The blood also brings white cells which clean up debris and secrete growth factors.) The end result is a scar. Dressings are changed regularly. During the period of healing, there would again be soreness, but severe pain would arise only in the event of infection.

Amputation

Amputation is one of two therapies that could be especially agonizing. While there is evidence of therapeutic amputation as long ago as 31,000 years, there is no consistent literature to clarify the indications and techniques involved [4]. If gangrene develops at the far end of a limb, it is necessary to amputate the limb above the gangrene, closer to the attachment of the limb to the body. (Gangrene usually occurs in the limbs and is due to a loss of blood supply either from injury or disease. Gangrene is initially dry, and the tissues gradually turn black. It is incurable and the gangrenous tissue must be excised, because otherwise it becomes infected, resulting in wet gangrene, which is hot, swollen, stinks, and is quickly lethal.) Amputation is the only treatment and, even with modern technology, is a major assault on the system. Hippocrates was the first to describe the principles underlying the need for amputation in cases of gangrene. He wrote:

> *When flesh, sinew, and bone are mortified, they are to be separated, and the parts which still live are to be preserved [5].*

Nonetheless, there is limited mention of surgery in the Hippocratic Corpus [6]. His treatment was conservative, and if all else failed, he would operate to facilitate separation of the diseased tissue at the gangrene–normal tissue interface. This might not have been as painful as one might imagine because, as pointed out by a later surgeon, the gangrenous tissue was insensible [7]. Celsus was the first to describe the technical details of surgery using modern principles. He cut the limb in a healthy place above the gangrene. The skin should be incised, and the soft tissues (muscles, tendons, nerves, and blood vessels) must be cut down to the bone and then pulled in the direction of the limb's attachment to the body. This would reveal the bare bone that should be sawn. The rough end of the bone would be smoothed. The skin must be shaped and mobilized enough to cover the bone end [8]. There was no mention of pain or pain relief in Celsus' text. However, his writings were lost until republication in 1478, so they had little influence until their rediscovery.

Lithotomy

The procedure of lithotomy was also described in some detail by Celsus. The word yet again comes from ancient Greek, where λίθος or lithos means stone and τομία or tomía means cutting. It was painful, and sadly Celsus had no suggestions on how to minimize the pain. Indeed, no efforts to reduce the pain of the procedure were made until the seventeenth century.

HUMAN PHYSIOLOGY AND PATHOLOGY FOLLOWING HIPPOCRATES

The treatments and their consequences described above are all related to observable physical phenomena. They are not much concerned with theories of body function. However, such theories would have an important impact on other aspects of medical management. Hippocrates (460 BC to c. 370 BC) was influenced by predecessors who were also concerned with the nature of matter. These included Alcmaeon (late sixth to early fifth centuries BC) and Empedocles (494 to 434 BC), whose ideas may have contributed to the contents of Hippocrates' essay, 'The Nature of Man'. In this seminal text, the notion of humours was propounded [9]. There were four:

blood, phlegm, yellow bile, and black bile. The different humours contributed to the personality, which would arise from the sum of the individual humours' contribution. Thus, blood was sanguine and hot and wet. Yellow bile was choleric and hot and dry. Black bile was melancholic and cold and dry, while phlegm was phlegmatic and cold and wet. If the humours were mixed in harmony, the patient was healthy; a condition called eucrasia. If the patient was sick, the humours were out of balance; a condition called dyscrasia. There were other factors which impacted on the balance of humours, such as seasons, diet, and astrology. The impact of these strange ideas would be hard to overemphasize, as it will become clear later and in subsequent chapters.

PAIN INFLICTED BY CAUTERY

The term cautery comes from the ancient Greek word καίεω, which means to burn.

Earliest Days

Cautery requires fire. It would seem fire became a routine component of human activity around 350,000 years ago, long before civilization and written records [10]. Cautery, which uses instruments heated in the fire, came much later. Mesopotamia, the first civilization with records of medical practice, was apparently unaware of cautery [11]. The first mentions of the practice were found in the Egyptian papyri. In the Ebers Papyrus, dated to 1550 BC, there is the following statement.

> *When thou meetest a tumour of the Vessels in any part of the body of a person and thou findest it round in form, growing under the finger, and spread out against the flesh; it is not big and does not protrude; then sayest thou: 'It is a tumour of the met. I will treat the disease. The metu causes it and it then becomes a pricking of the met'. Treat it with the knife and burn it with Fire so that it bleeds not too much. Heal it like the Cautery heals [12].*

In the Edwin Smith papyrus dated to 1650 BC, cautery is mentioned in Case XXXIX. The title of this case is 'Tumors or Ulcers of the Breast'. In the Breasted translation the condition is described as follows.

> *If thou examines a man having tumors with prominent head in his breast, (and) thou findest that the swellings have spread with pus over his breast, (and) have produced redness, while it is very hot therein, when thy hand touches him.' The proposed treatment for this condition is 'Thou shouldst say concerning him: 'One having tumors with prominent head in his breast, (and) they produce cists of pus. An ailment which I will treat with the fire-drill [13].*

The next mention is from Hippocrates whose final aphorism (LXXXVII) in section VII states:

> *Those diseases which medicines do not cure, are cured by the knife. Those that the knife does not cure are cured by fire. Those that fire does not cure, must be considered incurable [14].*

Cauterization and Its Effects on the Tissues

The heated implement burns the tissue, inducing a coagulation necrosis with inflammation and oedema [15]. (Necrosis is death of living tissue. Coagulation necrosis is a form of necrosis in which the dead tissue structure appears unchanged and the cell outlines can be seen under the microscope, although the nuclei are missing. It is caused when blood supply is blocked or by burns. Oedema is an accumulation of water in the tissues between the cells. This causes swelling and has two causes. In the first, in the absence of a blood supply, the walls of the small capillaries become more permeable, and fluid leaks out of the blood into the tissues. In the second, death of cells damages the cell walls, which also become more permeable, leaking fluid into the tissues. Both mechanisms occur with burns.)

Cutting with Cautery

If a cautery tip is fine and heated to a high temperature, it can be used to make precise incisions. This technique reduces the amount of bleeding from the margins of the incision.

Cautery and Haemostasis

Blood vessels are soft tubes, the walls of which include proteins (like collagen and elastin). When these proteins are denatured by heat, they shrink and fuse together, plugging the vessel mechanically and biologically. (Proteins have a complex folded structure. Denaturation is a process whereby this structure is destroyed and, since a protein's function relies on its shape, that function is lost.)

Heating infected material, such as a purulent discharge, can kill the bacteria in the discharge and thereby facilitate healing.

Cautery and Eschar Formation

Cautery has been used to induce eschar formation to prevent repeated dislocation of the shoulder [16]. (Eschars are pieces of dead tissue that have become hard and dry. They are often dark in colour with a crusty or leathery appearance. They most commonly develop after severe burns.) The use of eschar formation in the treatment of recurrent shoulder dislocations was described by Hippocrates [5]. The idea was that producing this tough material in front of the shoulder joint prevented the bone from being displaced forwards.

Cauterization and Issues

The term issue in the current context is unfamiliar today, but it is noted in Black's Medical Dictionary. The entry is:

> *Issue: is an old term for a suppurating sore [17].*

It is not found in the medieval texts but is mentioned once in Wiseman's writings [18]. Unsurprisingly it is Lorenz Heister who clarifies this term with the greatest cogency. He wrote:

> *Issues are little Ulcers made designedly by the Surgeon in various parts of the Body, and kept open by the Patient, for the Preservation or Recovery of Health [19].*

He goes on to describe their function and locations:

> *In this Operation the Physician endeavours by Art to imitate and relieve Nature, who often forms Ulcers in various Parts of the Body of her own accord, for discharging pernicious Humours, whereby People are often freed from grievous Disorders, and enjoy a healthy State. The Parts in which Issues are generally made, are either, (1.) the upper Part of the Head; (2.) the Neck; (3.) the Arms, betwixt the Biceps and Deltoeide Muscle, near the Insertion of the last; (4.) in the Thighs, especially within-ſide, immediately above the Knee, in a Cavity easily felt by the Fingers; and lastly, (5.) Issues are sometimes made in the Legs, on their interior ſide, in a Cavity immediately below the Knee [19].*

While this makes little sense today, it made sense when considered in relation to humoural concepts of physiology current at the time it was written.

As mentioned above, in the section on humoural physiology, humans were considered to have different temperaments based on the balance of the different humours. In this context, the various surgeons believed that different temperaments could affect the effectiveness of treatments, including cautery. Thus, Guy de Chauliac and William of Saliceto thought that it was less effective and possibly dangerous on people with a hot, dry temperament [20, 21]. The matter is most clearly stated by Albucasis, who wrote:

> *Now I say that the cautery has universal application for every ill constitution, whether organic or functional, with the exception of two: the functional hot temperament and the functional dry temperament. About the organic dry temperament the Ancients differed, some saying that cautery helps in a constitution of this kind, while others said the opposite: that cautery is of no use in a disease caused by heat or dryness; for fire is naturally hot and dry and it is obviously absurd to treat a hot dry sickness with a hot dry remedy. But he who holds the opposite view says that actual cautery may help in the case of such hot dry illnesses as arise in the human body; for when you compare the human body, humid as it is, with the nature of fire you find the human body cold. I myself from much experience agree with this last opinion [22].*

This quote is a splendid example of how humoural theory can be manipulated to suit any notions a given writer wishes to expound. Much later, in the Renaissance, Ambroise Paré [23] would point out that the elements were intellectual notions without physical form. On the other hand, the humours had physical form [22].

Since there was not one shred of evidence to support these theories, it may well be asked why they persisted. The answer is relatively simple. In any intellectually informed professional situation, the ideas that are generally accepted as true represent a safety net. If an individual diverges from the generally accepted norms, he/she will be at risk of criticism or punishment. Introducing new ideas is never easy. The Nobel Laureate Max Planck stated the progress of ideas very neatly:

> *A new scientific truth does not triumph by convincing its opponents and making them see the light, but rather because its opponents eventually die, and a new generation grows up that is familiar with it [24].*

COUNTERIRRITATION

There is one other application of cautery to be considered. It is easy to understand the use of the method to stop bleeding, incise a lesion, or burn necrotic tissue. However, it was also used in quite a different way to produce what is called counterirritation. Hippocrates' forty-sixth aphorism in the second book states

> *When two pains occur together, but not in the same place, the more violent obscures the other [14].*

Whether this was the stimulus that started the use of cautery to treat invisible targets with the aim of reducing pain at a distance is not clear. However, it does provide a conceptual basis for the use of cautery to relieve pain. Nearly four more centuries would pass before Celsus made his contribution to the method. He was not much concerned with the pain of cautery, making only a passing reference to it (see Chapter 3). It should also be noted that there were two types of cautery. Actual cautery involved burning the skin with a piece of heated metal, while potential cautery involved the use of caustic chemicals. While perhaps less dramatic, the potential cautery was widely regarded as inferior, as the distribution and extent of spread of caustic chemicals were not easy to contain.

Celsus was the first writer to outline specific uses of cautery. While most of his cases involved the treatment of visible lesions, there were already indications for symptoms without a visible target. This could at best treat symptoms rather than diseases. Moreover, not only was any notional benefit purely symptomatic, but it also involved the delivery of intense pain in a procedure incapable of therapeutic benefit.

How the procedure worked is unknown, although numerous unconfirmed theories have been proposed [25]. Figure 2.1 illustrates a multitude of sites for cautery applied to invisible lesions. The underlying reasons for choosing a particular location for such treatments remain obscure.

Cameron Gillies, the author of a book on counterirritation, was at pains to emphasize that treatments can be accepted if they are known to work, even if there is no understanding of the way they achieve their effect. A perfect example of this is the use of digitalis for the treatment of heart failure. Its function was discovered by William Withering and published in 1795 [26]. The mechanism of action of the drug did not become clear until the late 1960s. Thus, for close to 175 years, digitalis was prescribed without an understanding of its mechanism of action. This lack of understanding in no way minimized the value of the drug.

Gillies mentioned his personal experience, where counterirritation had often proved beneficial. He suggested a mechanism stating that:

> *The essential action of a counter-irritant is to quicken the circulation in the part to which it is applied and towards the point of application [27].*

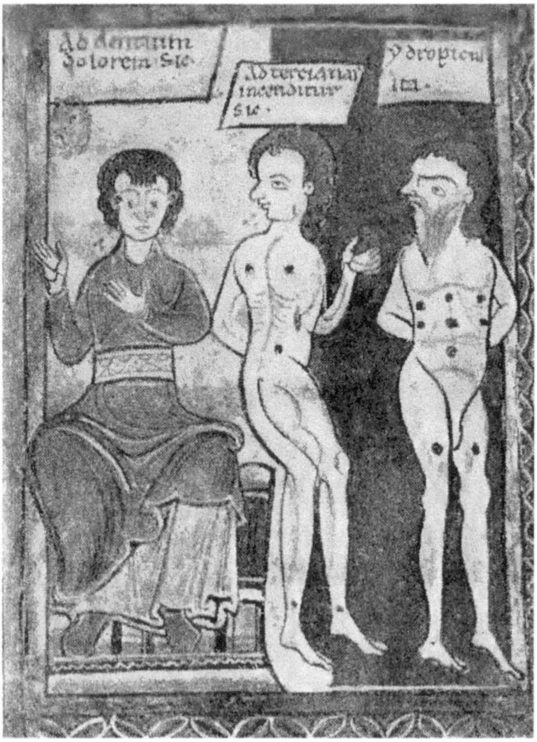

FIGURE 2.1 13th-century image.

Shows some places where cautery was applied for counterirritation.

The text continues with a number of examples of beneficial cautery, but nothing is presented that would be considered scientific evidence today.

CONCLUSION

Exposure to pain, whether from injury, illness, or therapy, was a consistent feature of surgical treatments down the centuries. Acceptance of this pain only makes sense if people were aware of the torments suffered by those who received no treatment. In the twenty-first century, we have little knowledge of the diseases suffered in the ancient world. However, in the eighteenth century, a number of surgical textbooks contained elegant illustrations drawn by talented surgeons, revealing exotic extremes of illness quite unknown in the twenty-first century. These fearsome images make it easier to understand the realities our forebears had to face and provide a basis for understanding why they would need a surgical professional who, while trying to heal them, would inflict so much agony.

REFERENCES

1. Ulmer BC. Electrosurgery: History and Fundamentals. *Perioperative Nursing Clinics*. 2007; 2: 89–101.
2. Paulo D, Semonche A, Choudhry O, Al-Mufti F, Prestigiacomo CJ, Roychowdhury S, et al. History of Hemostasis in Neurosurgery. *World Neurosurgery*. 2019; 124: 237–250.
3. Johnson T. *Of Wounds in Generall. The Workes of the Famous Chirurgion Ambroise Pare: Translated out of the Latine and Compared with the French*. London: Richard Cotes; 1649, pp. 252–255.
4. Maloney TR, Dilkes-Hall IE, Vlok M, Oktaviana AA, Setiawan P, Priyatno AAD, et al. Surgical Amputation of a Limb 31,000 Years Ago in Borneo. *Nature*. 2022; 609: 547–551.
5. Hippocrates. *On Joints. Hippocrates. III*. Cambridge, MA: The Loeb Classical Library, Harvard University Press; 1995, pp. 201–397.
6. Christopoulou-Aletra H, Papavramidou N. The Manifestation of "Gangrene" in the Hippocratic Corpus. *Annals of Vascular Surgery*. 2009; 23: 548–551.
7. Theodoric B. *Gangrene. The Surgery of Theodoric ca AD 1267 Book 2*. New York: Appleton-Century-Crofts Inc; 1955, pp. 36–38.
8. Celsus. *De Medicina*. Cambridge, MA: Loeb Library, Harvard University Press; 1938.
9. Hippocrates. *The Nature of Man. Hippocrates. IV*. Harvard: Loeb Classical Library; 1931, pp. 1–41.
10. Shimelmitz R, Kuhn SL, Jelinenk AJ, Ronen A, Clark AE, Weinstein-Evron M. 'Fire at Will': The emergence of habitual fire use 350,000 years ago. *Journal of Human Evolution*. 2014; 77: 196–203.
11. Majno G. *The Asu. The Healing Hand*. Cambridge, MA: Harvard University Press; 1965, pp. 29–68.
12. Ebers G. *Ancient Egyptian Medicine The Papyrus Ebers*. Chicago, IL: Ares Publishers; 1930, p. 148.
13. Breasted JH. *Case 39 Tumors or Ulcers in the Breast Perhaps Resulting from Injury. The Edwin Smith Surgical Papyrus*. Chicago, IL: Chicago University Press; 1930, pp. 363–369.
14. Hippocrates. *Aphorisms. Hippocrates Volume IV*. Cambridge, MA: Harvard University Press; 1931, pp. 97–221.
15. Kumar V, Abbas AK, Aster JC, Deyrup AT, Das A. *Robbins and Kumar Basic Pathology*, 11th ed. Philadelphia, PA: Elsevier; 2023.
16. Nayab M. History of Amal-i-Kaiyy (Cauterization) and Its Indications According to the Shapes of Instruments: A Review. *International Journal of Medical and Health Research*. 2017; 3(3): 60–61.
17. Macpherson G (Ed.) *Black's Medical Dictionary*, 39th ed. Lanham, MD: Madison Books; 1999. Issue.
18. Wiseman R. *Of Gun-shot Wounds in General. Eight Chirurgical Treatises*. London: Walthoe, J.; 1734, pp. 152–153.
19. Heister L. *Of Issues. A General System of Surgery in Three Parts. 1*. London: W Innys; 1743, pp. 314–316.
20. de Chauliac G. *The Major Surgery of Guy de Chauliac: An English Translation*. USA: Xlibris; 2007.
21. Saliceto W. *The Surgery of William of Saliceto*. USA: Xlibris; 2002.
22. Albucasis. Introduction. In *Albucasis on Surgery and Instruments - A Definitive Edition of the Arabic Text with English Translation and Commentary*. Berkeley, CA: University of California Press; 1973, pp. vii–xv.

23. Johnson T. *Of Elements. The Workes of the Famous Chirurgion Ambroise Pare: Translated out of the Latine and Compared with the French.* London: Richard Cotes; 1649, p. 3.
24. Planck M. *Scientific Autobiography and other Papers.* London: Williams & Norgate Ltd.; 1950.
25. Gillies HC. *Introductory. The Theory and Practice of Counter-Irritation.* London: Macmillan & Co.; 1895, pp. 1–15.
26. Rosner L. *Withering, William. Dictionay of Medical Biography.* 5. London: Greenwood Press; 2007, pp. 1315–1316.
27. Gillies HC. *The Uses of Counter-Irritation generally. The Theory and Practice of Counter-Irritation.* London: Macmillan & Co.; 1895, pp. 124–136.

3 Surgical Pain in the Ancient World

HIPPOCRATES CA. 460 BC – CA. 370 BC

Hippocrates was the first to report the techniques of surgery. His writings include mentions of surgical technique and a few notes on how the pain of surgery should be managed (Figure 3.1).

SURGERY

Hippocrates opens his remarks in the text called 'In the Surgery' with a short list of the requirements of surgery. The list comprises the patient, the operator, assistants, instruments, and lighting, with consideration given to the nature and location of the abnormality to be operated. The correct position of the hands and arms is specified, together with advice on the best way to stand or sit. Control of the movement of the

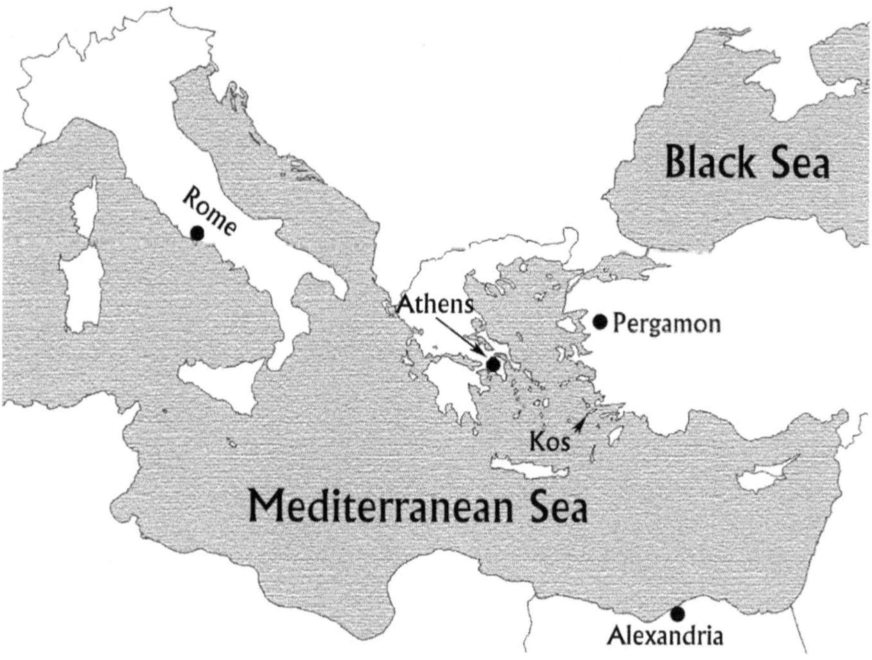

FIGURE 3.1 Important surgical centres of classical times.

DOI: 10.1201/9781003748816-3

hands is necessary, involving ambidextrous control. The aim is to achieve grace, speed, painlessness, elegance, and readiness [1]. This covers pretty much everything relevant to the efficient performance of a surgical operation. What matters in the present context is the need to minimize pain, about which he had further comments elsewhere in his writings. This need is expressed as follows.

> *In surgical operations that consist in incising or cautery, speed or slowness are commended alike, for each has its value. In cases where the surgery is performed by a single incision, you must make it a quick one; for since the person being cut generally suffers pain, this suffering should last for the least time possible, and that will be achieved if the incision is made quickly. However, when many incisions are necessary, you must employ a slow surgery, for a surgeon that was fast would make the pain sustained and great, whereas intervals provide a break in its intensity for the patients [2].*

Cautery

Hippocrates stated that there was a place for cautery in therapy. In his view it was to be used when all else had failed.

> *Those diseases which medicines do not cure, are cured by the knife. Those that the knife does not cure are cured by fire. Those that fire does not cure, must be considered incurable [3].*

Hippocrates also described how surgery and cautery could be combined in the same treatment, haemorrhoidectomy. That must have involved particularly intense agony [4].

> *First undertake to find out where the haemorrhoids are; for to incise the anus, to amputate from it, to lift it by sewing, to cauterize it, or to remove something from it by putrefaction – these seem to be dangerous, but in fact will do no harm. I bid you to prepare seven or eight irons, a span in length and the width of a wide probe; bend these at the end like a small obol [? spit ?]. Clean the site you are attempting to cauterize beforehand with a medication, have the person lie on his back, and place a pillow beneath the loins. Force the anus out as far as possible with your fingers; heat the irons red-hot, and burn until you so dry the haemorrhoids out that you do not need to anoint: burn them off completely... Let assistants hold the patient down by his head and arms while he is being cauterized so that he does not move – but let him shout during the cautery, for that makes the anus stick out more [4].*

The above passages outline, in a way readily understood in the twenty-first century, that Hippocrates was well aware of the suffering of patients, and attempted both to minimize it and, where suitable, to use it to advantage.

There is one indication for cautery which today seems almost eccentric, yet Hippocrates described it in great and precise detail. The Hippocratic method for reducing shoulder dislocations, using the heel of the foot as a fulcrum, is well known. The patient lay on his/her back. The surgeon's heel was placed in the armpit, and the arm was pulled outwards and upwards. The heel redirected the traction force onto the head of the humerus, causing it to glide back into position. [The bone of the upper arm is called the humerus. The head of the humerus is the round upper end of the bone, which forms part of the shoulder joint.) In addition to a description of how to reduce a shoulder dislocation, Hippocrates also made a thorough presentation of how to prevent recurrent dislocation of the shoulder. He introduced the topic with remarks about the importance of preventing recurrent dislocations, which could spoil a career in sports or result in danger on the battlefield. The technique was as follows:

> *One should cauterize these cases thus: Grasp the skin at the armpit between the fingers and draw it in the direction towards which the head of the humerus gets dislocated (i.e. downwards), then pass the cautery right through the skin thus drawn away. The cautery irons for this operation should not be thick nor very much rounded, but elongated (for so they pass through more quickly), and pressure should be made with the hand. They should be white hot, so that the operation may be completed with all possible speed. For thick irons, since they pass through slowly, leave larger eschars to come away, and there is risk of cicatrices breaking into one another [5].*

The use of white-hot irons does sound like torture. It is important to note that Hippocrates, like most later authors, thought that the shape of the actual cautery instrument should be adapted to suit the specific task for which it should be used.

Analgesics

There is no mention of the use of analgesics related to surgery. This was not because there were no analgesics available. Opium was familiar to Hippocrates, who mainly used it for gynaecological complaints, in particular the 'wandering womb', the term for which was hysteria [6].

CELSUS (CA. 25 BC – CA. 50 AD)

Surgery

Over three centuries later, Celsus had written a definition of the qualities required of a surgeon, which would come to be most influential many centuries later.

> *Now a surgeon should be youthful or at any rate nearer youth than age; with a strong and steady hand which never trembles, and ready to use the left hand as well as the right; with vision sharp and clear, and spirit undaunted; filled with pity, so that he wishes to cure his patient, yet is not moved by his cries, to go too fast, or cut less than is necessary; but he does everything just as if the cries of pain cause him no emotion [7].*

This is a sensible and sensitive passage, including the need for the surgeon to avoid distraction occasioned by the intensity of the patient's distress and to function as though he, the surgeon, had no emotion, even though this was not the case. With this description in mind, Celsus also wrote about the correct management of the pain of lithotomy, which, involving access via a route between the scrotum and the anus, must surely have been one of the most terrifying procedures. Bladder stones occur mainly in males. They are found in men around fifty years of age and in boys.

In Celsus material, the age range for surgery was between nine and fourteen years of age [8]. Bladder stones in children are found in low-resource countries. Their occurrence is related to temperature and food [9–11]. This would suggest that the diet of ancient Rome was less than optimal. Celsus wrote:

> *then the operation is carried out in a warm room, and in the following manner. A strong and well-trained man, seated on a high stool, seizes the boy from behind and draws him backwards until his buttocks rest on the man's knees. When the boys' legs have been drawn up, the man orders him to put his hands behind his knees, and to pull upon them as much as he can, and at the same time the man keeps them in this position. But if a stronger person is to be treated, two strong men are seated on stools, side by side, and both the stools and the adjacent legs of the men are lashed together, so that they cannot be separated. Then the patient is seated in the same way as above upon the knees of the two men; and according to their position, one man takes hold of the patient's left leg, the other of the right, whilst at the same time the patient pulls upon his own hams. Whether one or two men hold the patient, they press downwards with their chests upon the patient's shoulders [12].*

Thus, Celsus without any euphemism, clearly described the nature of a surgical procedure and how to cope with the difficulties. As outlined in Chapter 2, Celsus was the first to record an amputation through healthy tissue, closer to the attachment of the limb to the trunk than the gangrene requiring the operation. However, extremely painful though this must have been, there is no mention of pain or its management in the description of amputation.

Celsus showed that consideration of pain could influence the decisions he made when operating. He described two methods of treating a perianal fistula. One took a long time and was pain-free; the other was quicker but painful. The method chosen depended on the choices agreed between patient and surgeon. This is the only situation in De Medicina where a surgeon's decision relates to the pain of a procedure. In books seven and eight, which are concerned with surgery, all other mentions of pain are concerned either with the course of a disease or with post-operative healing. There is no other suggestion that pain should influence technique.

Regrettably, Celsus' wisdom would not become available to his successors until Tommaso Parentucelli, of Sarzana, discovered the manuscript to De Medicina in 1443 in a library in Milan. It was subsequently printed in 1478, the first medical text to be printed on Gutenberg's new printing press. Thomas went on to become Pope Nicholas V. The text of De Medicina which he had brought back under the light of day was to become most influential.

Cautery

Celsus mentioned the pain inflicted by cautery as related to the practicalities of treatment. Concerning the management of carbuncles he wrote:

> *The best thing is to apply a cautery at once; this is not a severe procedure, because the patient does not feel it, since the flesh is dead; and the cauterizing is stopped when pain is felt all over the lesion [12].*

Celsus advocated using cautery as a knife to incise the abdominal wall. He also used it to incise the wall of abscesses in the liver, carbuncles, abscesses in the limbs, and in the walls of the thorax. It was also used in the excision of cancers. There are conditions treated with cautery that sound alarming, including varices of the scrotum and penile warts. Even more disquieting is the recommendation to use a red-hot fine iron needle to reshape eyelids which have become inverted, a condition called entropion, which results in eyelashes scratching the eye. It could also be used when a weakened lower eyelid drooped outwards, failing to cover the eye, a condition called ectropion. In addition, he mentioned that using diathermy to treat chronic atrophic rhinitis was very painful. This was the only mentions of pain related to cautery in his writing.

Celsus also used locations for cauterization of normal skin in some treatments. These different indications required the application of the cautery in a location determined by the symptom being treated. The mechanism of action of treatments of this kind was not explained and remains obscure, although in some instances counterirritation, as mentioned in Chapter 2, might have played a role. While unlikely to provide any symptomatic benefit, it is fair to say that the choices of locations were often but not always close to the tissues which were intended to benefit from treatment. Thus, locations in the abdominal wall were used for flatulence and at the location of the pain for migraine. However, it is not easy to understand why epilepsy should have been treated by cautery to the back of the head close to the upper vertebrae. Nor is it easy to determine the logic of cauterizing the temples for patients with ophthalmia. (Ophthalmia is an inflammation of the eye and especially the conjunctiva. The conjunctiva is the membrane which covers the front of the eye and lines the eyelids.) There is again a reference of adapting the shape of the cautery to the local requirements.

Analgesics

Celsus was familiar with opium as an agent that could induce sleep and relieve pain. However, there is no mention of opium in any part of the text related to surgery.

Phlebotomy

Bloodletting to modern practitioners involves the removal of blood through an almost completely painless needle. The process takes less than a minute. Any reader of surgical history is familiar with the use of phlebotomy to remove blood with a view to recovering the balance between the humours (see Chapter 2). What is less considered is the duration and discomfort associated with the condition. This was noted by Celsus who wrote:

> *Now blood-letting, whilst it may be very speedily done by one practised in it, yet for one without experience is very difficult, for to the vein is joined an artery, and to both sinews. Hence should the scalpel strike a sinew, spasm follows, and this makes a cruel end to the patient [13].*

The consequence of neural or tendon injury as a result of phlebotomy will be seen to be a recurring issue in this book.

DIOSCORIDES (CA 40 AD TO CA 90 AD)

Analgesia

Dioscorides was born ten years before Celsus died. Moreover, he lived a century before Galen. He wrote the first pharmacology textbook with the title 'De Materia Medica'. In it he described the qualities of four plants with narcotic and analgesic properties. Henbane had many other properties but could be used as an analgesic given as suppositories. Hellebore was especially used as a purgative. However, it could also be used for epilepsy, depression, delirium arthritis, and paralysis. The opium poppy was of course used as an analgesic and to induce sleep. Then there was the mandrake, which Dioscorides classified as a poisonous narcotic. He wrote as follows.

> *They give out also that there is another sort called morion growing in shady places and around hollows, having leaves similar to the white mandrake but smaller (as it were), twenty centimetres long, white, lying round around the root. This is tender and white, a little longer than twenty centimetres, the thickness of the great finger. They say as much as a teaspoon of a decoction of this (taken as a drink or eaten with polenta in placetum, or food that is eaten with bread), will infatuate [cause unconsciousness]. For a man sleeps in the same fashion as when he ate it (sensible of nothing for three or four hours) from the time that it is brought him. And physicians also use this when they are about to cut or cauterize [14].*

To return to Dioscorides' suggestion that Mandrake could reduce the pain of surgery. It must be remembered that he was a botanist, not a physician/surgeon. Galen, who came later, had other ideas.

GALEN (CA 130 AD – CA 210 AD)

Pain of Surgery

Galen was prolix and wrote much, and there is a comprehensive translation into German by Karl Gottlob Kühn, but nothing equivalent in English. However, Dr. Christine F. Salazar's book 'The Treatment of War Wounds in Graeco-Roman Antiquity' has provided useful insights into Galen's approach to the pain of surgery [15, 16]. There are various quotations from the works of Galen illustrating his management of the pain of surgery. He was like any authoritative clinician interested in distinguishing fake pain from the real thing. As far as medicaments were concerned, the analgesics available to Galen, who lived a century after Dioscorides, were outlined above in the section on Dioscorides.

There is further awareness to be gained from a doctoral thesis from the University of Colorado, entitled 'Galen on Pain,' by Courtney Roby. Here it is mentioned that Galen considered the above-mentioned available anaesthetic remedies unsatisfactory and their use was plagued with potentially dangerous complications [17].

There is another issue. Goby mentions that it is unexpected that Galen showed so little interest in treatment focused simply on pain. However, Galen provides an explanation for his attitude in his Method of Medicine Book XII.7. He states as follows:

> *If we could eradicate the actual cause due to which patients suffer pain, we would be acting in this way, not against the symptom but curing the patient. However, when we are prevented for some reason from proceeding against the condition, we mitigate the severity of the pains [18].*

Thus, Galen, like many subsequent surgeons, considers curing the underlying pathological processes took precedence over relieving the discomfort resulting from these processes. He provided three case histories of men with colic. However, his reasoning and dietary treatments are so imbued with the notions of humoural pathology that they do not really contribute further to our understanding. One final text illustrates a humanity which is not normally associated with Galen. It is indirect evidence that he was emotionally affected by the pain inflicted by surgery. In his book on anatomical procedures in the part concerned with exposing the brain in the living animal he wrote as follows.

> *I say, then, that for this purpose you must procure either a pig or a goat... you avoid seeing the unpleasing expression of the ape when it is being vivisected [19].*

Otherwise, it may be noted that the mention of pain in Galen's animal vivisection is noteworthy for its absence [20].

Apart from the specific teachings on pain just mentioned, Galen was of supreme importance to the practice of medicine for centuries to come. As Vivian Nutton wrote:

> *...his ideas constitute the basis of formal medicine in Europe at least until the seventeenth century [21].*

Indeed the value of Galen's teachings was first questioned only as late as the Renaissance, where his statements on cranial anatomy began to be called into question [22]. His remarks about surgery are concerned with technique, and there is no suggestion that technique should be modified to reduce patient suffering.

Pain of Cautery

Galen was aware of a complication of cautery not previously mentioned. The procedure leads to the formation of dead tissue called an eschar (see Chapter 2), which in time separates from the underlying healthy tissue. According to Galen this separation could be accompanied by severe bleeding which might be difficult to treat [15].

Analgesia

While not enthusiastic about the use of soporific analgesics during surgery, Galen still found a use for them. They could be given to induce unconsciousness, thereby avoiding fainting due to pain, which he considered could end fatally [15]. However, this refers to the pain of disease. Galen was also familiar with opium [23], but again there is no evidence that he used it to reduce the pain of surgery [16].

Phlebotomy

Galen wrote extensively about phlebotomy, but his writing is concerned mostly with indications, location of venepuncture, and the expected results. He does, however, make two important comments related to technique. He instructed that changes in the pulse during bloodletting were a firm indication that the bleeding should be stopped [24].

In his 'Anatomical Procedures' Galen, having made one comment on an incompetent practitioner, proceeds to mention others, writing:

> *I pass by, for the present, all the mischief they have done in blood-letting, by [their] failing to understand the parts to be watched in each of the veins at the elbow, of which I have spoken also in my book De mortuorum dissectione [25].*

PAUL ÆGINATA (CA 625 – CA.690)

Pain of Surgery

In his translation of the works of Paul Æginata, Frances Adams remarked about book six that

> *This book contains the most complete system of operative surgery which has come down to us from ancient times [26].*

The value of these writings is confirmed by other authors. Harold Ellis, commenting on Paul's description of tracheostomy in 2009, wrote:

> *This description would well serve a modern textbook [27].*

In addition, Vivian Nutton wrote:

> *Paul's Book 6 is by far the most informative (and most practically minded) Greek surgical text extant [28].*

In Paul's Book 6 devoted to surgical topics, there is no mention of the pain of surgery. There is no mention of opium, the poppy, or mandrake. However, Paul's awareness of anxiety related to undergoing surgery is mentioned. There are two comments on patients who could not endure eyelid surgery, without a reason given for this. For the treatment of fistula in ano, Paul noted that timidity led some patients to refuse to an operation. This leaves the impression that acceptance of the pain of surgery was related to the courage of the patient. Pain relief was not considered applicable. Paul repeated the previously mentioned requirement of restraining patients who were to undergo lithotomy. Again, there is no mention of adapting technique to minimize suffering.

Pain of Cautery

Paul Ægineta thought highly of cautery [29] but was selective about its application. His texts were influential, and the use of cautery would be maintained in mainstream treatment for centuries to come. Some of his treatments would terrify any rational person. He advocated cautery for circumcision if the foreskin was diseased and also for hypospadias, the condition where the opening of the urethra is under the penis and further back than the tip. He also advocated its use in the groin and scrotum for hernias and hydroceles. (A hernia is a weakness in the wall of a body cavity, usually the abdomen, which permits contents to be extruded outside the cavity. A hydrocele is a fluid-containing swelling within the scrotum). More rational was the use of cautery to open the walls of pus collections, as advocated by Celsus. However, he had one most unusual indication. In cases of bite by a poisonous snake, he advocated excising the bitten portion and cauterizing the tissue bed left following excision.

Paul also used diathermy for invisible targets. Like Celsus, he treated ophthalmia, but the location he used was the vertex of the skull down to the bone, rather than the temples.

Paul Ægineta did mention the pain of cautery. With regard to vitiligo, he mentioned that patients avoided the treatment due to dread of the pain involved, which, from a modern point of view, would seem to be profoundly sensible.

Analgesics

Paul mentions ointments such as tetrapharmacon [30] or Egyptian ointment [31], which could be soothing on a wound. There is no mention of oral analgesia.

Phlebotomy

Paul mentions the universal use of phlebotomy but does not describe either the technique or the complications.

CONCLUSION

Hippocrates and Celsus, while describing the need for immobilization of patients during surgery, do not comment on the management of the pain as such. Paul Æginata mentions that it could happen that patients refused surgery, a decision which he attributed to timidity. It is clear from Hippocrates and Celsus that surgeons were aware of pain and the need for restraint. However, it is clear that the pain is part of the treatment and is to be accepted. Hippocrates mentions ways of minimizing pain by adjusting the speed of the surgery. Celsus and Galen disliked pharmacological analgesia because of the side effects of the drugs involved. Celsus alone comments not only on the stress of the patient but also on the strains suffered by the surgeon. He specified that being a surgeon meant that the distress of an operation should not be a reason for cutting short a procedure because of the patient's anguish.

There is reason to believe that pain was more accepted in Classical times. After all, many painful diseases, including cancers, were quite untreatable, and their development to a fatal conclusion had to be accepted. This was a time when fighting in battle involved hacking with steel weapons at individual enemies, face-to-face. Everyday conditions such as toothache, earache, backache, and rheumatic pain all had to be tolerated, as there were no means of alleviation. In such a milieu, it seems reasonable to suggest that, while unwanted, pain was not as unacceptable as it is today. It required less attention for its relief.

REFERENCES

1. Hippocrates. *The Surgery. Hippocrates. III.* Cambridge, MA: The Loeb Classical Library, Harvard University Press; 1995, pp. 53–81.
2. Hippocrates. *The Physician. Hippocrates. VIII.* Cambridge, MA: The Loeb Classical Library, Harvard University Press; 1995, pp. 297–311.
3. Hippocrates. *Aphorisms. Hippocrates Volume IV.* Cambridge, MA: Harvard University Press; 1931, pp. 97–221.
4. Hippocrates. *Haemorrhoids. Hippocrates. VIII.* Cambridge, MA: The Loeb Classical Library, Harvard University Press; 1995, pp. 377–385.
5. Hippocrates. *On Joints. Hippocrates. III.* Cambridge, MA: The Loeb Classical Library, Harvard University Press; 1995, pp. 201–397.
6. Inglis L. *The Ancient World. Milk of Paradise*. London: Picador; 2019.
7. Celsus. *Book VII, Proemium. De Medicina.* Cambridge, MA: Loeb Library, Harvard University Press; 1938. pp. 295–299.
8. Celsus. *Book VII, Part 6. De Medicina.* Cambridge, MA: Loeb Library, Harvard University Press; 1938, pp. 425–447.
9. Rizvi SHR, Sultan S, Zafar MN, Ahmed B, Umer SA, Naqvi A. Paediatric Urolithiasis in Emerging Economies. *International Journal of Surgery*. 2016; 36: 705–712.
10. Leslie SW, Sajjad H, Murphy PB. Bladder Stones. In *StatPearls*. Treasure Island, FL: StatPearls Publishing LLC.; 2025.
11. Skolarikos A, Jung H, Neisius A, Petřík A, Kamphuis GM, Davis NF, et al. Prevalence, Aetiology, and Risk Factors of Bladder Stones. In *EAU Guidelines on Urolithiasis*. Arnhem: Netherlands; 2025, pp. 69–70.
12. Celsus. *De Medicina*. Cambridge, MA: Loeb Library, Harvard University Press; 1938, pp. 125–175, 155–65, 425–47.
13. Celsus. *De Medicina*. Cambridge, MA: Loeb Library, Harvard University Press; 1938, pp. 155–165.
14. Dioscorides. *4-76. Mandragoras. De Materia Medica.* Johannesburgh, SA: Ibidis Press; 2000, pp. 624–627.
15. Salazar CF. *Surgical Aspects of Wound Treatment. The Treatment of War Wounds in Graeco-Roman Antiquity*. Leiden: Brill; 2000, pp. 9–53.
16. Salazar CF. *Pharmaka. The Treatment of War Wounds in Graeco-Roman Antiquity*. Leiden: Brill; 2000, pp. 54–67.
17. Roby CA. *Galen on Pain*. Ann Arbor, MI: University of Michigan; 2005.
18. Galen. *Book XII.7. Method of Medicine. Book XII.7.* Cambridge, MA: Loeb Library, Harvard University Press; 2011, pp. 283–299.
19. Galen. Exposure of the Brain in the Living Animal. In: Lyons MC, Towers B, editors, *Galen on Anatomical Procedures, The Later Books*. Cambridge, MA: Cambridge University Press; 2010, pp. 15–17.
20. Gleason MW. Shock and Awe: The Performance Dimension of Galen's Anatomy Demonstrations. In: Gill C, Whitmarsh T, Wilkins T, editors, *Galen and the World of Knowledge*. Cambridge, MA: Cambridge University Press; 2009, pp. 85–114.
21. Nutton V. The Fortunes of Galen. In: Hankinson R, editor. *The Cambridge Companion to Galen*. Cambridge, MA: Cambridge University Press; 2008, pp. 355–390.

22. Da Carpi B. *Fracture of the Skull or Cranium*(Translation). Philadelphia, PA: The American Philosophical Society; 1990.
23. Africa TW. The Opium Addiction of Marcus Aurelius. *The Journal of the History of Ideas*. 1961; 22(1): 97–102.
24. Brain P. *On Treatment by Venesection. Galen on Bloodletting*. Cambridge, MA: Cambridge University Press; 1986, pp. 67–99.
25. Galen. *On the Care Needed in Investigating Nerves and Vessels. Galen on Anatomical Procedures*. Oxford: Oxford University Press; 1956, pp. 81–82.
26. Ægineta P. *Preface to the Surgical Part. The Medical Works of Paulus Aegineta, The Greek Physician*, Translated into English. London: The Sydenham Society; 1834, pp. 247–248.
27. Ellis H. *The Dark Ages and the Renaissance. The Cambridge Illustrated History of Surgery*. Cambridge, MA: Cambridge University Press; 2009, pp. 22–34.
28. Nutton V. *Medicine in the Later Roman Empire. Ancient Medicine*. 2nd ed. London and New York: Routledge; 2013, pp. 299–317.
29. Adams F. *Seven Books of Paulus Ægineta*. London: The Sydenham Society; 1846.
30. Adams F. *On Plasters, and Those Things Which are Added to the Boiling of Them, from the Works of Antyllus, and On the Proportion of Wax to Oil. Seven Books of Paulus Ægineta. 3*. London: The Sydenham Society; 1846, pp. 558–580.
31. Adams F. *On Different Preparations of Oil and Ointment. Seven Books of Paulus Ægineta. 3*. London: The Sydenham Society; 1846, pp. 589–598.

4 Surgical Pain – Middle Ages

INTRODUCTION

At any time, disease is protean and evolving. Its defeat depends on knowledge for the treatment of what is known and research to discover more of what is not known. Medicine requires theoretical and practical components. The medicine of the ancient world, as propounded by Hippocrates and expanded by Galen, included both practice and theory. It was written in Greek. The Roman Empire became too large to administrate from a single centre. In 286 AD, the Emperor Diocletian divided it into two provinces, West and East. Not long after this, in 313 AD, the Emperor Constantine the Great published the Edict of Milan, granting tolerance to Christianity within the Roman Empire. In 380 AD, Theodosius published the Edict of Thessalonica, which proclaimed the form of Christianity based on the Nicene Creed to be the official form of the religion within the empire. He was the last emperor of the entire empire. Thereafter, in 395 AD, the empire was formally divided into two empires, with two emperors: western and eastern. The religion of the western empire was Roman Catholicism with Latin as its language, and the religion of the eastern empire was Greek Orthodoxy, with Greek as its language.

Nearly a century after the split of the empire, the Western Empire collapsed in 476 AD. While Rome diminished as a political centre, it remained the main focus of the expanding Roman Catholic Church, the dominant component of Christian administration [1]. While the language of the Christian administration was Latin, most medical writings of importance were in Greek, the primary language of the eastern empire. In Europe, education and educational institutions increasingly came under the influence of the Church. Medical teaching used limited Latin translations of Hippocrates and Galen. What information was acceptable depended on the approval of the church. There was a widespread notion that the health of the body was of secondary consideration. What mattered was the health of the soul [2]. While there might have been a few doctors in the cities, there was a marked lack of educated health care outside them [1]. This lamentable state of affairs persisted for several centuries.

In Byzantium, recent medical texts consisted of encyclopaedias describing accepted medical knowledge. These systematic encyclopaedias were learned, organized, and practical, but they were not original [1]. The learning they contained together with texts of Hippocrates and Galen were to emigrate into the Arab world, where they would be enriched by such authorities as Rhazes and Avicenna.

In Europe, the first event which marked a return to academic surgery, interested in theory as well as practice, was the work of Abu Al-Qasim Al-Zahrawi, widely referred to as Albucasis. He was an Arab physician who lived and worked near Cordova in Spain (see Figure 4.1).

DOI: 10.1201/9781003748816-4

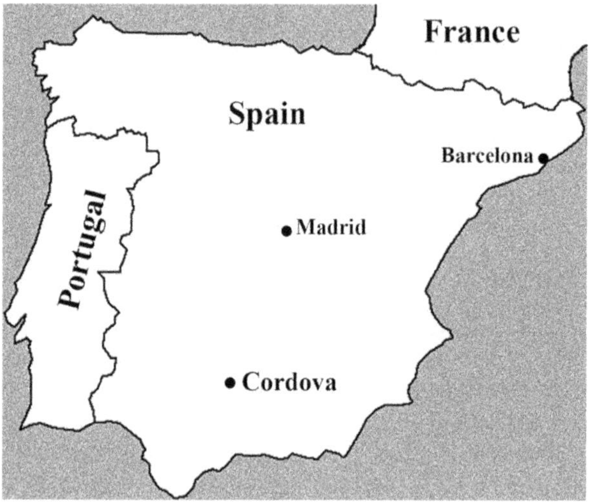

FIGURE 4.1 Outline map of Spain.

Showing location of Cordova.

ABŪ AL-QĀSIM KHALIF IBN -AL'ABBĀS AZ-ZAHRĀWĪ (ALBUCASIS) (936 TO 1013)

Albucasis, who wrote in Arabic in the tenth century, based his writings for the most part on Paul Ægineta's work. Thus, the guidelines of medical knowledge remained the works of the classic period, in particular those of Hippocrates and Galen. In the ancient world, medicine was a skill learned by apprenticeship [3].

Albucasis was the first to lament the fall in social status of surgeons. The book was the first text devoted to surgery alone. He explained that the lowly position of contemporary surgery was due to the lack of proper theoretical and practical training, as expressed in the opening paragraphs of his mighty book '*Albucasis on Surgery and Instruments*.' He wrote:

> *For the skilled practitioner of operative surgery is totally lacking in our land and time; so that the knowledge of it is on the point of being blotted out and its remains lost; and there is nothing left of it except a few traces in the books of the Ancients; where, however, it has been so corrupted by the hands of scribes, and subjected to error and confusion, that its meaning has become obscured and its value diminished. Therefore I decided to revive this art by expounding, elucidating, and epitomizing it in this treatise; and to present the forms of the cauterizing irons and other operative instruments, since this is an adjunct to explanation and a vital necessity [4].*

It has been reasonably considered that the loss of status was also due to the changes in the profession of surgery as it developed during its sojourn in Arab lands. It has been suggested that oriental fatalism, religious proscription of touching the dead, and timidity in the face of haemorrhage were all factors that contributed to the decline of the status of the profession [5]. As an Arab, Albucasis had access to the translations of Greek texts from earlier times, and his work, as mentioned, is largely based on the writings of Paul Æginata [6].

Pain of Surgery

Albucasis makes no mention of methods to alleviate the pain of surgery, but he does refer a number of times to changing techniques to accommodate the desires of nervous patients. With regard to abdominal warts, he wrote:

> *On the other hand if you see that the patient is frightened and dreads the cutting of them with the scalpel, take a wire of stout lead, and ligature this type of wart and leave for two days. Then increase the stricture by the lead wire and go on doing this as it sinks into the wart, until the wart is cut through and spontaneously falls away with no trouble [7].*

With respect to the circumcision of boys, he uses various methods to reduce the youngster's anxiety as follows:

> *The manner of operating is first to make the boy, especially if he is one who understands a little, imagine that all you are going to do is tie a ligature on the tip of the penis and leave it for another day. Then amuse him and cheer him up as much as you can, according to his intelligence; then stand him upright before you, not sitting; and hide the scissors in your sleeve or under your foot and do not let the boy's eye chance upon that or any other instrument [8].*

With regard to the management of hydroceles, he wrote:

> *If the patient be timid and will not suffer the operation on account of its unpleasantness, then treat by perforation as I shall now describe [9].*

And finally, there is the matter of piles:

> *But with the patient who refuses excision with the knife, this manner of removal should be practiced: thread a twisted thread into a needle, then draw the piles upward and run the needle through the root of each, from one side to the other, and wind the ends of the thread round beneath the needle as it lies crosswise, and bind the pile firmly; then knot the thread and remove the needle. Do this with each pile, but leave one not destroyed so that superfluous blood may flow from it. Then apply to the anus a piece of material soaked in oil of roses or wax; apply it and bid the patient lie quiet; then leave him until the piles fall away [10].*

These various remarks indicate an awareness of patient anxiety and a willingness to accommodate it. However, there is the clear understanding that such anxiety is the result of nervousness, and while there are no direct judgemental statements about the quality of this anxiety, there remains an impression that it is the result of weakness.

Finally, Albucasis mentions that relevant parts of patients' bodies had to be immobilized for cranial cautery, tooth extraction, extraction of a dead fetus, scrofula resection, and cautery to a lachrymal fistula.

Pain of Cautery

Albucasis' account of cautery is the most comprehensive of any of the medieval surgical writers. It includes details of instrumentation and technique not to be found elsewhere. He used it for loose teeth and toothache. He continued in the tradition of using it to prevent recurrent shoulder dislocation. In addition, he used it for inguinal hernias. However, there is no mention of its use for lesions of the penis or scrotum. On the other hand, his finding cautery appropriate for the removal of corns and the haemostasis of the bed of an excised wart suggests over-enthusiasm. The use of it for gangrene, cancer, and the haemostasis of a bleeding artery makes more sense.

On the other hand, Albucasis advised cautery for far more invisible targets than any other surgeon. Fully two-thirds of Albucasis' cauterizations were for counterirritation and not for the direct effect of heated metal on visibly sick tissue. It is not necessary to repeat the exhaustive list of indications. However, the following illustrates well the weakness of the concepts governing treatment. A lesion over the frontal bone in the midline was used for apoplexy and epilepsy, as well as other indications. In cases of phlegmatic lethargy, lesions could be placed again in the frontal prominences, the middle of the head or the occiput. Lesions for hoarseness and dyspnoea were placed at the throat or the junction of the neck with the last vertebra. Lesions for pleurisy were located between the neck and the clavicle, below the jugular veins and at the nipples. Haemorrhoids were treated with lesions over the umbilicus, lumbar region, and liver. Diarrhoea was treated with lesions around the umbilicus, in the lumbar region and over the coccyx. Urinary incontinence was treated with lesions around the navel, in the pubic hair, and in the lower part of the back. There were other absurdities, but the list is long enough to make the point.

Analgesia

Albucasis makes no mention of medication to relieve pain. His extensive use of cautery would indicate that he was comfortable with inducing pain in a good cause. No predecessor had been comfortable with analgesic medicine. Since he tried to relieve anxiety by changing technique, it would seem he was humane.

Phlebotomy

Albucasis warns about the risk of injuring a nerve when taking blood from the median vein of the arm. He does not mention pain but states that the consequence of such an injury is stupor, which could be fatal [11].

LATE MEDIEVAL LEARNING

Academic surgery became re-established in Europe in the twelfth century, just over a hundred years after the death of Albucasis. Albucasis, being an Arab, had full access to the Arabic translations of the texts of the Ancient World, mainly those of Hippocrates, Galen, and Paul of Ægina. In addition, he could read the texts written originally in Arabic by such as Rhazes and Avicenna. Such learning was not available to other practitioners without translations. Moreover, even if they had been available, the texts of the old masters would have remained inaccessible, since the language of European academia and that of the new universities which began to be founded at this time was the Latin of Christianity. Thus, what was required were translations into Latin. This would have been a formidable task because while the material included ordinary language, the medical literature also contained a vast number of technical terms. In addition, the manuscripts that came to be translated would possibly have been written after the text had been processed by generations of copyists. Thus, there were many potential sources of error. Apart from translation, every manuscript was published by making copies, which again introduces the possibility of error. Moreover, many of the historical manuscripts, still available in museums, while ancient, may yet be copies produced long after the original. Having stated the need for caution when interpreting these translations, there is yet no denying their importance for the development of medicine and surgery in the Middle Ages. The first of these translators came from what is now Tunisia, and his name was Constantine.

Constantine the African (ca.1017 to ca.1087)

This gentleman was a Saracen (Muslim) merchant [12]. He is thought to have come from Ifriqiyah, a region equivalent to western Libya, modern Tunisia, and eastern Algeria. The capital was Kairouan. Constantine travelled widely, collecting medical literature. On visiting Salerno, a significant centre of medical learning just over forty-five kilometres south-east of Naples, he discovered there was no Latin medical literature. In consequence, he returned home to Ifriqiyah for three years and studied. He then returned to south Italy and joined the Monte Cassino monastery close to Salerno, with its excellent library. It was there that he undertook his work converting Arabic into Latin. Constantine translated only Arabic texts into Latin. It seems that these were the only two languages with which he was conversant [13].

Gerard of Cremona (ca. 1114 to 1187)

There is very little available about this gentleman's life. It is said that Gerard travelled to Toledo searching for scientific knowledge, particularly information about the astronomer Ptolemy. He translated seventy-one Arabic texts into Latin [14]. These included twenty-four works on medicine. His translations included Avicenna's Canon, which would be the prime text on medicine until the late seventeenth century. He also translated the surgical parts of the writings of Albucasis.

Salerno

The re-emergence of academic medicine in Europe was a concomitant of certain social changes. These were the above-mentioned translation of ancient texts, the rise of urban centres and the formation of universities [3]. These did not arise in a vacuum

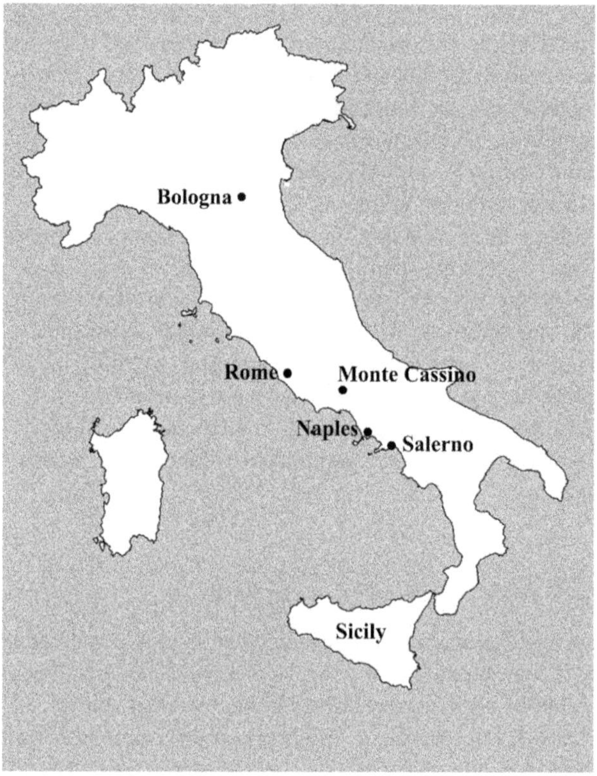

FIGURE 4.2 Outline map of Italy.

Showing Italian surgical centres.

but had mostly evolved from existing schools, which the church had taken over [15]. After all, at this time, most learning in Europe was an ecclesiastical monopoly. Medical schools began to appear (see Figure 4.2), where surgeons with updated ideas about their craft published new texts.

They were influenced by the translations of classical texts by such workers as Constantine and Gerard mentioned above. However, there was a new sense of innovation, and these surgeons were motivated to demonstrate that surgery was a science requiring the book learning of its principles as well as manual skills. Thus, they each wrote a textbook of surgery considered more up to date than anything published previously [16]. Their writings could reasonably have been expected to tackle the problems resulting from the pain of surgery, but some ignore the problem, while others approach it at best tangentially.

ROGER FRUGARD OF PARMA (1140 TO 1195)

There is nothing known of Roger's family, training, and upbringing. His book is laid out systematically, proceeding to discuss ailments and injuries starting in the head and proceeding down the body to the feet.

Pain of Surgery

Roger makes no allusion to the management of pain related to the surgeon's knife. On the other hand, he introduced a new method of investigating cranial trauma, which would have reduced patient suffering. It was considered important in those days to determine if a traumatic cranial fissure affected the entire cranial thickness, or whether it was limited to the external layers of the skull. The traditional way of determining the thickness of a fissure was to instil ink into the fissure and then scrape inwards. If the ink was no longer visible before the scraping had penetrated the full thickness, then nothing further needed to be done. If the fissure was full thickness, then it would have been necessary to undertake a trepanation. Frugard suggested that the patient should perform a Val Salva manoeuvre. (Breathing out forcefully while keeping the mouth closed). If the fracture was full thickness, material would seep out through the fissure. If it was partial thickness, nothing happened. This method of determining fissure depth, saved patients from a lengthy and painful open operation.

Apart from avoiding unnecessary pain, Frugard has several mentions of patient restraint. These are mostly related to realigning parts of the skeleton that have been either dislocated or fractured. However, there are two situations where the patient is immobilized prior to surgery. For goitre surgery, the patient was restrained by being tied to the table before the operation began. Moreover, for lithotomy, the patient was immobilized in a suitable position by a 'sturdy' assistant. These may reasonably be considered immobilization to prevent the pain-induced movements resulting from the procedure to be undertaken. Despite the availability of opium, there is no mention of its use to reduce the pain of surgery.

Pain of Cautery

The different indications for cautery are much fewer than those mentioned by Albucasis, but again, Roger's book is much shorter than that of his predecessor. He also used the treatment for invisible indications, but visible lesions comprise the majority of cases treated. In terms of pain, there are three mentions of patients refusing cautery because of the agony involved. In all three cases, cautery is refused because of the fear of the patient. Alternative treatments were offered. In one case, the knife was used instead of the cautery. In the other two, the alternative treatment was the use of caustic ointments. It is interesting that the author made allowances for the pain of cautery but made no such mention with respect to the use of the scalpel. Again, opium is not mentioned as an analgesic with respect to cautery [17].

Analgesia

Roger introduced a new ointment called Apostles or Apostolicon. This promoted healing and relieved pain [18]. He also advocated the inhalation of fumes from heating garlic and henbane to relieve the pain of toothache [19].

Phlebotomy

There is no comment on the technique of phlebotomy and its possible complications.

ROLAND OF PARMA (SPECIFIC DATES NOT KNOWN)

Less is known about Roland than about any other surgeon of his time. There is a record that he assisted Hugh of Lucca in Bologna during pulmonary surgery. It is not certain where he trained. His book, known as the 'Rolandina' contains much of the contents of Roger of Parma's book.

Pain of Surgery

There are mentions of immobilizing patients during lithotomy and surgery for goitre. There are no mentions of managing pain induced by the knife.

Pain of Cautery

There is no mention of pain in relation to cautery. In Roland's material, indications for cautery were slightly more frequent for counterirritation than for direct cauterization of sick tissue.

Analgesics

There is no mention of opium used for analgesia [20].

Phlebotomy

There is no comment on the technique of phlebotomy and its possible complications.

BRUNO DA LONGOBURGO (CA 1200 TO 1296)

A little more is known about Bruno than his predecessors. He was born in Longoburgo, a small town in Calabria in southern Italy. It is possible that he spent time in Salerno. It is also possible that he may have studied with Hugh of Lucca in Bologna together with Theodoric (see below). At all events, he ended up practicing in Padua, in the eastern part of the Po valley in northern Italy. He was familiar with the works of earlier surgeons, quoting Galen, Avicenna, and Albucasis amongst others.

Pain of Surgery

Bruno mentions again the need to restrain patients who were to undergo lithotomy. There is no mention of restraint for thyroid surgery. On the other hand, the sequence in surgery of inguinal and scrotal hernias is first to reduce the hernia in the standing patient and mark the region to be operated. The patient then lies supine on a table to which he is bound, again presumably to prevent pain-induced movements. It is also noted that some patients preferred to suffer from medical treatment-resistant TB glands of the neck than to permit surgery, due to fear of the knife. In this case, a caustic ointment was applied as an alternative to the lancet. A similar fear applied to haemorrhoidectomy. In that case, the haemorrhoid was ligated and allowed to slough off.

Pain of Cautery

Bruno mentions more indications for cautery than either Roger Frugard or Roland, but still fewer than Albucasis. Nowhere is there any mention of pain preventing this treatment method. He cauterized a few patients for counterirritation.

Analgesics

Once again, analgesics such as opium are not mentioned as a means of reducing the pains of surgery.

Phlebotomy

There is no comment on the technique of phlebotomy and its possible complications.

THEODORIC BORGOGNONI (1205 TO 1298)

Theodoric is thought by some to have been the son of Hugh of Lucca mentioned above. He certainly had the greatest respect for Hugh, who is mentioned repeatedly in his writings. While nothing is known of Theodoric's personal biography, there is some information gleaned from his appointments and his own writings. He was an ordained Dominican friar who became the suffragan bishop of Cervia and also a confessor to Pope Innocent IV. His association with Pope Innocent IV meant he was close to some of the major political events of his lifetime. At the time of Innocent IV's election to the papacy in 1243, there was a long-standing conflict between the Holy Roman Empire and the Papacy. The Emperor Frederick II had been a pioneer of improving educational standards, including the study of medicine. He had been King of Naples and established standards of training in surgery at Salerno, which were superior to anything else available at that time [21, 22]. This same Frederick, as Emperor, insisted on '*imperialis potestas*', the unlimited right of the emperor to exercise autocratic power. The papacy, on the other hand, insisted on '*universalis potestas*', the church's claim to universal power. These two irreconcilable notions were termed the 'Investiture Controversy' and had led to the previous pope Gregory IX excommunicating Frederick II. Innocent IV, who did not trust Frederick II, retained the excommunication and, fearing for his life, fled to France in 1244, only to return home in 1250 following the death of Frederick II [23]. A confessor to the pope during such troubled times would have been well informed about public matters and perceived to possess considerable authority.

The organization of his text is systematic and divided into four books. The first book is concerned with the various traumatic conditions that may require surgery. The second book applies these principles by region, starting with wounds, proceeding to fractures and finishing with dislocations.

The text is discursive. He also gives an indication of his sense of superiority as expressed in the following text.

> *And anyone who reads carefully that book which I entitled 'The Daughter of the Prince' will be able by following the authority of the ancients, and the clearest reasoning, and this present doctrine, to refute a large measure of those things which have been written in the surgical texts of the moderns. But still I fear that we are ploughing in the sands, because they will not withdraw from their errors; for it is difficult to relinquish the things to which one is accustomed; and perhaps it is better to let those who are in error to continue to err in their own stupidity [24].*

Despite this overweening arrogance, Theodoric's text gives more attention to coping with the pain of surgery than any previous surgeon.

Pain of Surgery

Theodoric accepted that patients could be too frightened to accept an operation in a variety of circumstances. Treatment of fistulae was one source of such anxiety. (A fistula is an abnormal connection between two epithelial surfaces. Epithelium is a type of tissue that forms continuous sheets of cells, covering the external surfaces of the body, like skin, and lining the internal organs and body cavities, like the gastrointestinal system from mouth to anus or the airways from windpipe to alveoli. Alveoli are tiny air sacs of the lungs which allow for rapid gaseous exchange of oxygen inwards and carbon dioxide outwards.) Operations on fistulae could be undertaken with either a knife or diathermy. If the patient would not allow the use of a blade to widen the opening, then probes of wood or reeds could be used. If both the knife and cautery were refused, Theodoric specified enlarging the fistulous passage with a plant root. If the knife was refused for abscesses, or tuberculous glands in the neck, caustic medicines should be used. With haemorrhoids, ligatures were recommended if surgical excision was not accepted. The need for physical restraint to keep the operating field stable was outlined for scrotal, ventral, and inguinal hernias and also for lithotomies [25, 26].

Pain of Cautery

Theodoric used cautery frequently. About half the indications involved visible targets, while half were for counterirritation. He also noted a fear of cautery for fistulae. If the patient feared the fire, caustics could be used [26].

Analgesics

It has been mentioned repeatedly that the surgeons of the ancient world viewed opium with concern.

Theodoric mentions the use of analgesics twice and is thereby the first of the surgeons to consider the need to minimize the pain of surgery. In a section on skull contusions without wounds, he wrote about the ingestion of analgesics

And you should know that certain surgeons are overanxious to operate upon the wounded. In order to eliminate the sense of pain they use analgesics, a thing which I do not approve at all, because, since it is impossible to apportion the medication accurately in accordance with the condition of the wounded any such patients receive somniferous medicine and sink into the deep sleep of death [27].

This is eminently sensible, reflecting the fact that precision methods of producing drugs with identifiable, reliable, and consistent dosage were not available [28].

In another place, he wrote about the 'soporific sponge.'

The composition of a savour to be made by surgeons, according to Master Hugo, is as follows: take of opium, and the juice of unripe mulberry, hyoscyamus, tile juice of spurge flax, the juice of leaves of mandragora, juice of ivy, juice of climbing ivy, of lettuce seed, and the seed of the lapathum which has hard, round berries, and of the shrub hemlock, one ounce of each. Mix these all together in a brazen vessel and, then put into it a new sponge. Boil all together out under the sun during the dog days, until all is consumed and cooked down into the sponge. As often as there is need, you may put this sponge into hot water for an hour, and apply it to the nostrils until the subject for operation falls asleep. Then the surgery may be performed and when it is completed, in order to wake him up, soak another sponge in vinegar and pass it frequently under his nostrils [29].

It should be noted that the sponge delivered analgesics without inducing the dangers concomitant upon ingestion. It will be seen later that opiates were considered suitable in ointments for painful lesions.

Thus, Theodoric, who on occasion expressed himself in a regrettably unsympathetic manner, was yet the first person to write about analgesia for the pain of surgery.

Phlebotomy

There is no comment on the technique of phlebotomy and its possible complications.

WILLIAM OF SALICETO (1210 TO 1277)

William was born in Saliceto, a village in northwest Italy. He studied at Bologna, and was a contemporary of Hugh of Lucca, Theodoric, and Lanfranc. He was considered to be the best surgeon amongst them. He insisted that an operation was not synonymous with surgery, which should be practiced with knowledge and ethics [30]. He was also regarded as superior by Malgaigne [31].

He defined surgery as follows:

Surgery is a science that teaches the principles behind the procedures for manual operations on the soft tissues, nerves and bones. We should not believe that any particular

manual operation constitutes surgery. But Surgery is a special body of knowledge that is not only a product of the mind; its objectives are clearly indicated and defined within indivisible and unalterable limits [32].

Pain of Surgery

William was a kind man, yet he was authoritative enough to insist that the patient should not contradict the surgeon. He made a number of references expressing his concerns over the suffering inflicted on patients during surgical operations and tried to modify his treatments to minimize the suffering. He insisted on manipulating the tissue as painlessly as possible. He was more gentle with feeble patients. In thigh wounds, deep drains were avoided as they could come into contact with unseen nerves and cause very bad pain. He avoided passing needles through nerves as this was agonizing. During trepanation, he blocked the ear canals in the mistaken belief that this would reduce the noise of drilling. Finally, he approved of the use of topical analgesics early in the management of wound pain. Saliceto again noted the need to immobilize patients undergoing lithotomy. He also recommended restraint for patients operated on for a direct inguinal hernia. [33]

Pain of Cautery

William of Saliceto made a comment concerning the use of direct cautery for a visible lesion. He took the treatment of cancer as an example. He states:

The actual cautery may cause a lot of pain just at the time of use, but overall it causes less suffering than cauterization with corrosive medicaments [34].

Actual cautery referred to the use of heated metal for cauterization as outlined in Chapter 2,which also referred to potential cautery, which is the use of corrosive medicaments. Interestingly, he used direct cautery to visible lesions in over two-thirds of his patients. He was seemingly less impressed with the technique of counterirritation [33].

Analgesics

Like Theodoric, William of Saliceto approved of the parenteral use of analgesics, but with a rather different methodology, as noted in the following two remarks. The first concerns pain from a wound:

Pain can be relieved by using narcotics. such as opium. henbane. poppies. Populeum,[1] ointment. etc. made into plasters and ointments and applied as defensives. The narcotics must not be used for long periods; they are to be prescribed against pain early in the case. If continued too long the damaged part will cool. will mortify and deteriorate and die. Therefore, limit them to brief courses and for severe pain [35].

For the second, concerning an abscess, he wrote:

> *When an infection first appears and produces pus and the suffering is intolerable, make use of the familiar defensive ointment with added opium, henbane and white poppies and lay it on thickly around the wound until the pain eases. Do not use it for too long; return soon to the ordinary defensives without the stupefacients [36].*

His recommended course of treatment with opium is refreshingly modern, even if the underlying understanding was based on humoural physiology rather than the understanding current in modern times.

Management of the Pain of Surgery

As noted, William made an effort to reduce the pain of surgery. He also made a remark that illustrates the differences in behaviour between his time and the present. It is relevant to repeat and emphasize, there were no simple, easily available analgesic tablets. Christians in William's time were expected to endure pain and suffering with humility to escape a worse ordeal in purgatory after death. The Church taught that pain during life was, in part, atonement for sin [2, 37, 38].

As mentioned initially, William emphasized the importance of the authority of the surgeon. Following introductory remarks on the need to behave in a seemly, civilized, and dignified manner, once a surgeon is accepted as the person in charge of management, the patient should not disagree with the surgeon but should accept his proposals without demur. This is stated as follows:

> *The patient should not contradict the surgeon at work with his own opinions nor should he interrupt him during his operations. In so doing he will cause the surgeon to be hesitant and to question his own knowledge. He will become fearful and tremulous, indecisive in everything, and the operations will be defective. The physician's efforts will be impeded and a curable patient may become incurable, or his illness will be aggravated and prolonged. Therefore, once he has chosen him to do the job, the patient should abide by the dictates and the methods of the surgeon. Those are the best conditions for a cure, and the result will favour both the patient and the surgeon [32].*

It seems reasonable to assert, given the very different social circumstances, as outlined above, that Salicet's insistence on authority could have contributed to the patient's acceptance of the unavoidable pain.

Phlebotomy

There is no comment on the technique of phlebotomy and its possible complications.

GUIDO LANFRANCHI (CA 1250 TO CA 1306)

It is thought that Lanfranc was born in Milan, to which he returned after being trained in Bologna by William of Saliceto. He was caught up in the persisting Investiture

Controversy, siding with the Guelph party, which supported the pope. Unfortunately, Milan was ruled by Galeazzo Visconti, who was of the party of Ghibellines, which opposed the pope, and they were successful. In consequence, Lanfranc had to flee Milan to Lyon in France. In 1295, he arrived in Paris, where he established a school of academic surgery, based both on knowledge of the literature and experience in the operating theatre.

His book starts with an exhortation to modesty and professional loyalty and dignity, similar to that in the book of his teacher, William of Saliceto. He makes very little reference to the pain of surgery.

Pain of Surgery

In one situation, he notes that painful treatment should be avoided for conditions which were untreatable [39]. In another, he advocates the use of opium-containing ointments for persistent pain in wounds [40]. He also recommended opium-containing ointments could be applied to persistently painful haemorrhoids. There are many places where he recommends oil of roses for wound pain [41]. It may be noted that modern work suggests that rose oil can be an effective analgesic, but more work on humans is still required to be certain [42].

Pain of Cautery

According to Lanfranc, Avicenna had a high regard for cautery, but in the Italy of his day, it had fallen out of favour, not least because it was used by ill-educated practitioners with improper technique. It is worthy of note that nearly three-quarters of his indications were for counterirritation, not direct application to a visible lesion.

Excellent surgeon and academic though Lanfranc was, his contribution was more in the spread of the teachings of his master rather than the contribution of new notions.

Analgesics

There is no mention of analgesics for reducing the pain associated with surgery.

Phlebotomy

There is no comment on the technique of phlebotomy and its possible complications.

HENRI DE MONDEVILLE (1260 TO 1320)

Henri was born into what was the little village of Mondeville (see Figure 4.3). It has since been absorbed into the expanding city of Caen in northwest France, of which it is now a suburb. He studied in Montpellier and Paris to become a Master of Medicine. He then studied in Bologna under Theodoric. He clearly prospered because the first mention of him in a document lists him as one of the Royal Surgeons assigned to Montpelier, where he taught Medicine, Surgery, and Anatomy. While a

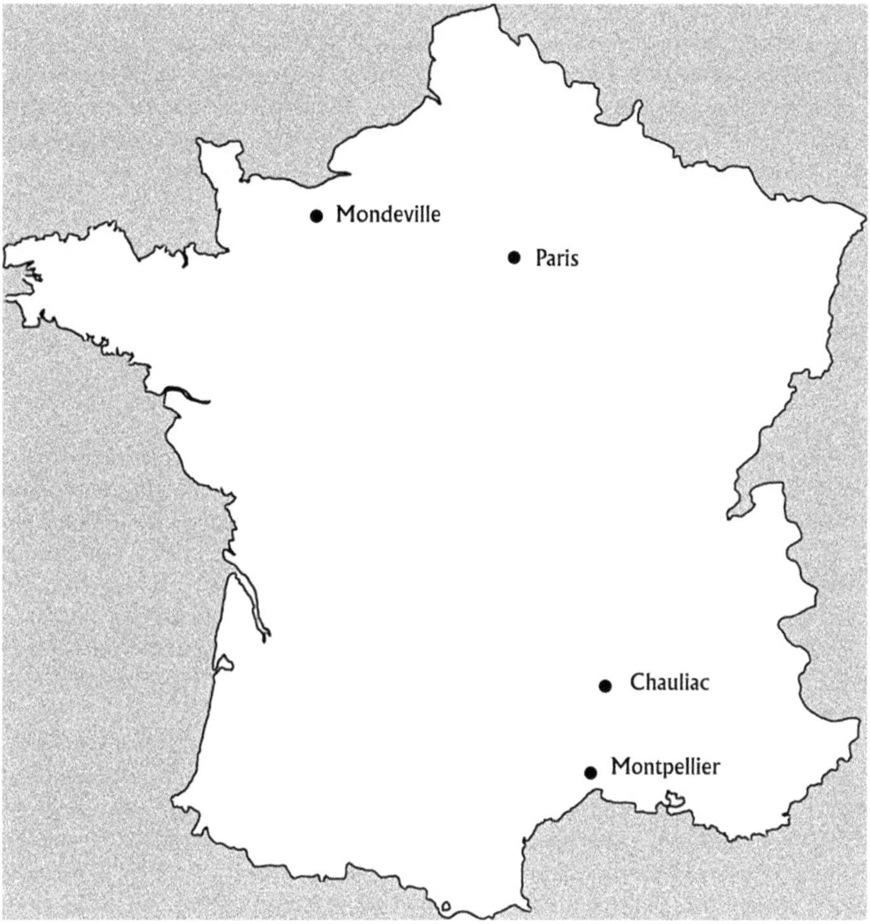

FIGURE 4.3 Outline map of France.

Showing French surgical centres.

distinguished honour, the Royal appointment became an annoyance over time, as it was not accompanied by any form of emolument [43].

Henri was outspoken and critical of those in authority, including the priesthood and royalty. His belief in the importance of his profession is perhaps encapsulated in the remark that:

> *God Himself practised surgery when he molded man from the primal mud, and when he created Eve from a rib, and when he made a plaster from a whiff of dust and spittle and rubbed it over the eyes of a blind man and restored his vision. Those miracles and many more like them and even greater, as are written in the Divine Book, were performed by God with his own hands. Nowhere is it written that he palpated the pulse of sick people or examined their evacuations and their urines [44].*

More than any of the other medieval surgeons, he reveals his passions, with on occasion amusing, irreverent comments on the use of alcohol by both patient and surgeon. He loved to set up lists. There is a set of principles governing the behaviour of surgeons, patients, assistants, and their interactions. Then there are notables, which are statements of the general principles of surgery. Moreover, there are contingents that relate to the details which govern practical management in individual cases.

Pain of Surgery

More than any prior author, Henri is aware of the pain inflicted by the surgeon's knife. There are a number of illuminating remarks.

> *All invasive surgical procedures do some harm to the involved member [45].*

He also made numerous comments indicating his wish to minimize pain. He advised gentleness with timid patients. Exhausted patients should avoid painful procedures. In feeble patients, a gentle touch was needed. It was noted that pain was better tolerated when the patient was in the company of friends [46]. He further insisted that assistants should follow certain rules of behaviour. They should remain calm and agreeable. They should not quarrel or mutter. They should not reveal the content of the surgeon's opinion and approach. The reason for these proscriptions was that they prevented activities that could alarm, scare, or disturb patients. There are no details of immobilization techniques.

Pain should be avoided when treating children, the faint-hearted, and the weak-minded [47]. In particular, the probing of wounds favoured by old-fashioned surgeons should be avoided, since it was so painful [48]. He states in two situations that surgery causes suffering [46, 49]. There are more remarks in the second volume of Henri's textbook, concerned with the treatment of specific diseases. There are several occasions in the text where patients refused the use of the knife [50–55].

Management of the Pain of Surgery

Henri de Mondeville reveals an approach that is similar to that of William of Saliceto. He emphasizes the unequal relationship between patient and surgeon, where the patient requires a service which the surgeon is in a position to deliver. He wrote:

> *Patients should heed their surgeons in all matters relevant to their diseases, neither in opposition to the operations or the advices [56].*

In addition, he seems to have had strict notions regarding the behaviour of patients. Although, as mentioned above, he was concerned with reducing the pain of surgical operations, nonetheless, he described patients who refused treatment as cowards; the only translation of the work of these medieval surgeons to use that term. It is found twice in the principles governing the use of actual cautery [57]. It is mentioned again with regard to bloodletting. De Mondeville suggests cowardly persons should be offered bread soaked in wine, syrup, or sugar of roses. Finally, the term is used as part of a more light-hearted section concerned with the interaction of alcohol and patients with surgeons. Of the surgeon, he wrote:

> *For example, he should never perform a serious operation such as making a large incision after he has been drinking. He should do that only when he is sober, especially when he operates on highly placed persons. There are seven exceptions:*
>
> > *When the urgency for action is great, as in treating fractures of the arm or dressing a fresh wound, even after the surgeon has imbibed his usual.*
> > *His hands tremble only slightly after he has had his usual weak morning quaff.'*
> > *If the lesion stinks, as with erysipelas or putrid gangrene, etc.*
> > *If he is an indecisive sort of weakling who needs a little weak wine to give him the courage to act.*
> > *If he worries that the patient will seek out another surgeon.*
> > *If he worries that he will have to refund a prepayment.*
> > *If he thinks that he must operate as soon as a reluctant patient consents, he who had consented after a period of indecision and may again change his mind.*
>
> *The reason why a surgeon should avoid operating after he has had his wine is that a bad result, even for any other cause unrelated to the drinking, will lead to an imputation that the fault was in the surgeon who was drunk when he operated. However, in those seven cases (above) the surgeon may operate, sober or not. But there are many more reasons to operate only when patients are sober, with one exception.*
> *Usually a sober patient's humors (i.e. digestive juices in this case) are more tranquil and are ready to flow when the time comes for him to eat. The exception is the enfeebled, cowardly and terrified patient who may come to a bad end if he is subjected to any operation when he is sober [58].*

This passage emphasizes the authoritative view a surgeon felt he was entitled to take in respect of his patient. Moreover, while de Mondeville was concerned about the spiritual weakness of cowardice, he also reveals a greater acceptance of material weakness related to the consumption of ethanol.

Pain of Cautery

Like Lanfranc, Henri favoured the application of cautery for counterirritation. Just under twenty per cent of the indications mentioned involved burning visible pathology. He was aware of the pain involved and advocated soothing ointments immediately after performing cautery [50, 51]. He does indicate his attitude to the refusal of cautery in the following remark:

> *Never use a caustic if you can find another way to do what is necessary and is tolerable for the patient. If he is not cowardly or unwilling to accept the hot instrument... [59].*

Analgesics

There is no mention of the use of analgesics to reduce the pain of surgery.

Phlebotomy

Henri de Mondeville opens his remarks on phlebotomy by stating that a physician decides if it is necessary. Then a surgeon should perform it. However, because it was simple to do and did not pay well, it had increasingly been undertaken by barbers. He states that a phlebotomist must have good eyesight and be able to avoid injury to adjacent arteries and nerves. With regard to complications, he notes:

> *Be careful when you open the cephalic vein not to prick the tendon that lies beneath it.... When you bleed from the basilic vein. avoid the artery which lies beneath it [52].*

He does not comment on how he would treat either of these complications.

JEHAN YPERMAN (CA 1260 TO 1331)

Yperman was born in 1260. He was educated in Latin and could study at the University of Paris, where he was taught by Lanfranc. He was married in 1285 to a lady who must have been a patient wife, because he studied under Lanfranc in Paris. Since Lanfranc arrived there in 1295, Yperman had already been married for around ten years, and his wife had had to tolerate the poor conditions of students in the big city [60]. After completing his studies, he returned to his native town, Ypres in Flanders. There, he was employed as a salaried surgeon at the city hospital. He was also expected to accompany the town's militia on military campaigns. In 1327, he was appointed doctor to the sick poor of the town [61].

He wrote a text on surgery, which returned to the structure of the text written by Roger of Parma. There are seven books starting at the head and proceeding downwards. Each book begins with regional trauma and then proceeds through a catalogue of non-traumatic conditions. Pages 41 to 173 are concerned with the neck and structures above it. That is 134 pages. The rest of the book consists of three codices, one from Brussels, one from Cambridge and one from Ghent. These deal with a variety of surgical conditions, not arranged with the strict organization of the first six books. These various topics from below the neck are covered in just eighty-eight pages, suggesting that Yperman was most interested in the surgery of the head and neck. However, what marks this book out from the remaining surgery texts of the period is that it is written in Flemish for Yperman's son, who knew no Latin.

Pain of Surgery

There is scant reference to the pain associated with surgical intervention. The one relevant comment relates to the shape of incisions. Yperman wrote:

> *If you can manage to treat the abscess without a cruciate incision, using only a linear one, you will obtain a cure with less pain and with a smaller scar [62].*

He was also the first of these surgeons to recommend washing hands before operating [63]. For patients who would not permit exploration of wounds, Yperman suggested the use of poultices [64].

Pain of Cautery

There is no mention of the management of the pain associated with cautery.

Managing Patients

Early in his book, Yperman lists sixteen ways of behaviour which should characterize a surgeon. There is no mention of the personality or behaviour of patients. The essence of his recommendations is listed below. It was of the very highest standard.

1. *He must be healthy in both mind and body.*
2. *The surgeon should have graceful hands and slender fingers and a sturdy frame that has no tremors. He should have sharp vision and be able to think clearly. He must be able to react promptly and unwaveringly.*
3. *Galen said that he must be modest and yet be courageous in his works.*
4. *The surgeon should be broadly educated beyond the realm of medicine.*
5. *He must not be a libertine. Rather he should maintain sobriety and chastity.*
6. *His religious faith should be beyond question.*
7. *He must devote himself completely to his patients,*
8. *When he is in the patient's home he will not disclose in any details that are related to his treatment, nor dally at length with the housewife, her daughter nor her servants.*
9. *I advise that he not make small talk with anybody because he may not know that the badinage may be offensive to the listener.*
10. *Do harm to none. Treat honorably all other surgeons and clergymen and express no envy of their successes.'"*
11. *He should not flatter himself.*
12. *He should have a serious mien and seek to earn a good reputation.*
13. *He should not offer a cure for a serious illness when there is no hope for success.*
14. *He will always offer solace to the patient.*
15. *He will state the condition clearly and accurately when the prognosis is very bad.*
16. *As to fees: he will take recompense according to the patient's financial means. He will treat the poor gratis.*

Despite the quality of his principles in the list, Yperman makes no mention of pain.

Analgesics

There is no mention of the use of analgesics to reduce the pain of surgery.

Phlebotomy

There is no comment on the technique of phlebotomy and its possible complications.

GUY DE CHAULIAC (CA 1300 TO 1368)

Guy de Chauliac was born in a small village in the diocese of Mende in the province of Auvergne in south central France. He was ordained, and his medical and surgical education was in Toulouse, Montpellier, and Paris. He also studied surgery in Bologna. He came to practice in Avignon at the time when the papacy was moved there, and he was one of the chaplains of three popes. He was better read than any previous surgeon [65]. He contributed little new, but he organized what was known in an outstanding manner. He was at pains to deprecate the way surgery to its disadvantage had been separated from medicine; a state of affairs he laid at the door of Avicenna. He gained great respect because he did not leave his post during the horrors of the Black Death.

De Chauliac persisted in the belief that the surgeon's relationship with his patient was authoritarian. He is required to be gracious with patients, generous with friends and wise with prognoses. On the other hand, the patient must follow the surgeon's instructions, much as the peasant obeys his feudal seigneur [66].

Pain of Surgery

De Chauliac was very aware of the need to immobilize patients during procedures. He finds it necessary for more indications than any other surgeon. He recommended it for the removal of arrows [67], amputation [68], tooth extraction and tonsillectomy [69], and lithotomy [70]. For hernia operations, patients were bound to the table [71]. Restraint was also necessary for such delicate procedures as removing redundant eyelashes or cataract removal [72]. He also registered that patients would refuse surgery because of anxiety [73–75].

Pain of Cautery

De Chauliac had relatively few indications for cautery. On the other hand, nearly two-thirds were for counterirritation and only a minority for the direct cauterization of visible pathology. He registered that not all patients could tolerate cautery [76].

Analgesics

In contrast with all his predecessors, de Chauliac recommended the use of opium ointment in a number of situations. These included wound pain [67], painful nasal ulcers [77], painful haemorrhoids [78], painful amputation [68], and painful toothache [79]. He describes the use of a soporific sponge, vapours from which could be inhaled by the patient, inducing sleep [68], as described by Theodoric [29].

In addition to these various indications, he mentioned that some surgeons permit opium by mouth. He has this to say about that:

> *Other surgeons have the patient drink opium; that is a dangerous action, especially for the young. I have heard that sometimes the patient becomes combative and savage, or manic, and sometimes dies [68].*

That is a statement consistent with the conventional wisdom passed down from classical times.

Phlebotomy

When describing the qualities of a phlebotomist, de Chauliac wrote:

> *He will grasp the knife with two or three fingers and will gently incise the vein. He will not penetrate or transect it, nor will he injure a nearby artery or nerve [80].*

MEDIEVAL MANAGEMENT OF THE PAIN FROM SURGICAL INTERVENTION

None of the surgeons mentioned in this chapter took the pain of surgery to be a major concern. They acknowledged its existence and, in addition, noted that certain patients found it intolerable. However, the writings leave the impression that the pain, while unpleasant, was something that should be accepted and tolerated with minimal complaint. Obviously, it could lead to unwanted movements during surgery, which were managed by immobilizing the patient either using assistants or by attaching the patient to the underlying furniture during a surgical procedure. A slight increase in the will to dampen surgical pain is seen in the later writings, where the use of narcotic analgesics was permitted during surgery, provided they were not taken by mouth. In addition, Lanfranc noted cautery was falling into disfavour because of its use by incompetent persons. Guy de Chauliac also recorded that not everyone could tolerate it. Moreover, it must not be forgotten that the authoritarian relationship expected by the surgeon would have the corollary that the patient, once having chosen a surgeon, would seek his approval. A component of that approval would involve the patient facing up to the necessary pains induced by treatment. Finally, all the surgeons whose work is considered in this chapter were university-trained, academics who wrote in Latin, with the exception of Yperman, even though there is evidence he went to university courses in Latin. These were surgeons of what would to be called the long robe, academically qualified, familiar with Latin and in many cases ordained. This was a pattern that would change after the Black Death.

CHRISTIANITY AND PAIN

In Chapter 1, it was noted that the health of the soul should take precedence over the health of the body, described by a text called the Ancrene Riwle, which was contemporary with the period described in this chapter. The text presented the notions that pain arising by chance was a test by God which should be endured, and that illness arising from irresponsible behaviour was a punishment requiring God's forgiveness. There is no statement consistent with this ideology in any of the surgical texts evaluated in this chapter. Nonetheless, God was important, of course, not least because healing required the help of God.

THE BLACK DEATH – AN AGENT FOR SOCIAL CHANGE (1345 TO CA. 1840)

The plague of the fourteenth century would have profound social consequences, not least on the practice of surgery, as will be related in subsequent chapters. For this reason, there follows a brief account of the aftereffects of the plague. One of the first parameters to determine is the actual number of people who died and the proportion of the population they represented. There is no consensus on this figure but the Encyclopaedia of the Black Death, while mentioning the difficulties in acquiring an accurate number [81], quotes Philip Ziegler, who suggested one-third of the population of Europe died. That would be in the region of 25,000,000 people [82].

It is not surprising that such a calamity could lead to exceptional social reactions. Two such popular changes in behaviour are commonly mentioned. The Flagellants were peripatetic groups who wandered around whipping themselves as demonstrative punishment for the sins that had brought the Black Death down upon the Earth [83, 84]. This is another, albeit eccentric, piece of evidence of how pain was tolerated in the past. It was not just a bizarre reaction to fear. It permitted the wider spread of the contagion because the Flagellants wandered about Europe to spread their messages, thereby facilitating the spread of the disease. The other commonly acknowledged unpleasant social reaction was the persecution of the Jews. This is, however, not relevant to the current narrative. There is, however, a third reaction which has received much less attention and yet might well have far more significant consequences. In disasters, an intuitive reaction is to support and help other family members. This is exemplified in an article called 'The Family and Disaster,' quoted below:

> *Disaster victims do not act as independent individuals, but their responses are to a high extent influenced by the families where they belong. Family members try to meet as soon as they learn that a disaster has occurred or is impending; they return to home if possible or they go to a place where they are likely to find other members of their families, often in the homes of relatives or close friends. Victims take great risks when they search for and try to rescue their family and kin, and it is almost impossible to keep them off a disaster site if they fear that family members are left in the debris. The same risk- taking can be seen before an impending disaster when people return to a threatened area to meet and look for their families [85].*

It is impossible for us to imagine the terror of a helpless population facing an impending certain painful death against which there was no remedy. Two contemporary authors described a reaction within families, which is most unusual. Boccacio in his Decameron relates the abandonment of infected patients by family and loved ones [86]. Guy de Chauliac also mentioned the same horrifying phenomenon:

> *They were very contagious, especially those who coughed blood, spreading the disease to those who lived near them as well to those encountered by chance. The dying patients were left alone, without servants or priests. A father did not attend his son, and the reverse. Charity was non-existent, and Hope was struck down [87].*

After the Black Death, the smaller population resulted in a fundamental change in social relationships. Landowners still needed the produce of their land, but the smaller number of tenants meant that these could negotiate better pay and conditions. In due course, a prosperous middle class developed, and the relationship between different social groups became more a matter of negotiation and less a matter of the unanswerable authority of those at the top of society [88]. Other changes also occurred with the passage of time, which may also relate to the disappearance of feudalism. Not only social but also academic authority became more and more subject to challenge, which in turn would affect the relationship between physician and patient. The beginnings of these changes will be included in Chapter 5.

NOTE

1 Populeum = Feather Moss

REFERENCES

1. Nutton V. Medicine in Late Antiquity and the Early Middle Ages. In *The Western Medical Tradition*. Cambridge: Cambridge University Press; 2009, pp. 71–87.
2. Rawcliffe T. Diseases of the Soul. In *Medicine and Society in Later Medieval England*. Stroud: Sutton Publising; 1995, pp. 1–28.
3. Temkin O. Medical Education in the Middle Ages. *Journal of Medical Education*. 1956; 31(6): 383–92.
4. Albucasis. *Albucasis on Surgery and Instruments - A definitive edition of the Arabic Text with english Translation and Commentary*. Berkeley, CA: University of California Press; 1973.
5. Zimmerman L, Veith I. *Albucasis [Eleventh Century] and the Surgery of the Arabic Period. Great Ideas in the History of Surgery*. New York: Dover Publications; 1967, pp. 81–92.
6. Albucasis. Introduction. In *Albucasis on Surgery and Instruments - A Definitive Edition of the Arabic Text with English Translation and Commentary*. Berkeley, CA: University of California Press; 1973, pp. vii–xv.
7. Albucasis. On the Amputation of Warts Occurring on the Belly. In *Albucasis on Surgery and Instruments - A Definitive Edition of the Arabic Text with English Translation and Commentary*. Berkeley, CA: University of California Press; 1973, p. 374.
8. Albucasis. Of the Circumcision of Boys; and the Correction of Their Erroneous Treatment. In *Albucasis on Surgery and Instruments - A Definitive Edition of the Arabic Text with English Translation and Commentary*. Berkeley, CA: University of California Press; 1973, pp. 396–400.
9. Albucasis. On Opening a Watery Hernia. In *Albucasis on Surgery and Instruments - A Definitive Edition of the Arabic Text with English Translation and Commentary*. Berkeley, CA: University of California Press; 1973, pp. 424–33.
10. Albucasis. On Cutting and Incising Piles that are Bleeding and the Treatment of Fissures. In *Albucasis on Surgery and Instruments - A Definitive Edition of the Arabic Text with English Translation and Commentary*. Berkeley, CA: University of California Press; 1973, pp. 512–5.
11. Albucasis. On Venesection. In *Albucasis on Surgery and Instruments - A definitive edition of the Arabic Text with english Translation and Commentary*. Berkeley, CA: University of California Press; 1973, pp. 624–55.
12. McVaugh M. *Constantine the African 2019*. Available from: https://www.encyclopedia.com/science/dictionaries-thesauruses-pictures-and-press-releases/constantine-african

13. Green M, Long B. *Constantinus redivivus: Reclaiming a Forgotten Cultural Translator 2018*. Available from: https://constantinusafricanus.com
14. Knight J. *Gerard of Cremona: 1114 - 1187 2018*. Available from: https://www.encyclopedia.com/people/philosophy-and-religion/philosophy-biographies/gerard-cremona
15. Malgaigne JF. *Thirteenth Century: Origin of the Universities-the Teaching and Practice of Surgery. Surgery and Ambroise Paré*. Oklahoma: University of Oklahoma Press; 1965, pp. 17–22.
16. McVaugh M. *The Rationalization of Wound Treatment. The Rational Surgery of the Middle Ages*. Firenze: Sismel, Edizioni Dedl Galluzzo; 2006, pp. 89–134.
17. Frugard R. *The Chirurgia of Roger Frugard Translated from the Latin Venetian Edition of 1546: XLibris*. Bloomington, IN: XLibris; 2002.
18. Frugard R. Proud Flesh (Grantulation Tissue) on the Dura Mater. In *The Chirurgia of Roger Frugard. 1*. Bloomington, IN: XLibris; 2002, p. 36.
19. Frugard R. Toothache. In *The Chirurgia of Roger Frugard. 1*. Bloomington, IN: XLibris; 2002, p. 66.
20. Parma R. *The Surgery of Roland of Parma*. Bloomington, IN: XLibris; 2002.
21. Nutton V. *Medieval Western Europe 1000 - 1500. The Western Medical Tradition*. Cambridge: Cambridge University Press; 2009, pp. 139–205.
22. Ghosh SK. Human Cadaveric Dissection: A Historical Account from Ancient Greece to the Modern Era. *Anatomy and Cell Biology*. 2015; 48(3): 153–69.
23. Guerello F. *Innocent IV*. 2024. Available from: https://www.britannica.com/biography/Innocent-IV
24. Theodoric B. *Wounds Anywhere in the Body*. In *The Surgery of Theodoric ca AD 1267 Book 2*. New York: Appleton-Century-Crofts Inc; 1955, pp. 137–9.
25. Theodoric B. *The Surgery of Theodoric ca. AD 1267 Book 1*. New York: Appleton-Century-Crofts Inc; 1955.
26. Theodoric B. *The Surgery of Theodoric ca. AD 1267 Book 2*. New York: Appleton-Century-Crofts Inc; 1955.
27. Theodoric B. Contusions of the Skull without Scalp Wounds. In *The Surgery of Theodoric ca AD 1267 Book 2*. New York: Appleton-Century-Crofts Inc; 1955, pp. 116–8.
28. Ng R. History of Drug Discovery and Development. In *Drugs: From Discovery to Approval*. Hoboken, NJ: Wiley-Blackwell; 2008, pp. 391–7.
29. Theodoric B. The Soporific Sponge and Sublimates. In *The Surgery of Theodoric ca AD 1267 Book 2*. New York: Appleton-Century-Crofts Inc; 1955, pp. 212–4.
30. Saliceto W. Dr Pifteau's Preface. In *The Surgery of William of Saliceto an English Translation*. Bloomington, IN: XLibris Corporation; 2002, pp. 21–31.
31. Malgaigne JF. Surgeons of the Thirteenth Century: Roger-Roland-Brunus-Théodoric-Guillaume de Salicet. In *Surgery and Ambroise Paré*. Oklahoma: University of Oklahoma Press; 1965, pp. 22–32.
32. Saliceto W. Preamble to Book I. In *The Surgery of William of Saliceto*. Bloomington, IN: XLibris; 2002, pp. 32–7.
33. Saliceto W. *The Surgery of William of Saliceto*. Bloomington, IN: XLibris; 2002.
34. Saliceto W. Cancers and Herpetic Esthiomene and Others. In *The Surgery of William of Saliceto*. Bloomington, IN: XLibris; 2002, pp. 74–6.
35. Saliceto W. Puncture Wounds of Nerves. In *The Surgery of William of Saliceto an English Translation*. Bloomington, IN: XLibris Corporation; 2002, pp. 135–9.
36. Saliceto W. Wounds of the Upper Arm. In *The Surgery of William of Saliceto an English Translation*. Bloomington, IN: XLibris Corporation; 2002, pp. 113–6.

37. Porter R. What is Disease? In: Porter R, editor. *The Cambridge History of Medicine.* Cambridge: Cambridge University Press; 2006, pp. 71–102.
38. Bourke J. Religion. In *The Story of Pain.* Oxford: Oxford University Press; 2014, pp. 88–129.
39. Lanfranc. The Requirements in the Manners and the Skills of the Surgeon. In *The Surgery of Lanfranchi of Milan.* Bloomington, IN: XLibris; 2003, pp. 32–6.
40. Lanfranc. Wounds in Nerves (ie Sinews). In *The Surgery of Lanfranchi of Milan.* Bloomington, IN: XLibris; 2003, pp. 45–8.
41. Lanfranc. *The Surgery of Lanfranchi of Milan.* Bloomington, IN: XLibris; 2003.
42. Mohebitabar S, Shirazi M, Bioos S, Rahimi R, Malekshahi F, Nejatbakhsh F. Therapeutic Efficacy of Rose Oil: A Comprehensive Review of Clinical Evidence. *Avicenna Journal of Phytomedicine.* 2017; 7(3): 206–13.
43. de Mondeville H. The Biography of Henri de Mondeville. In *The Surgery of Henri de Mondeville. 1.* Bloomington, IN: XLibris; 2003, pp. 61–70.
44. de Mondeville H. Notable XII The Three Methods of Treatment. The Superiority of Surgery. In *The Surgery of Henri de Mondeville. 1.* Bloomington, IN: XLibris; 2003, pp. 221–5.
45. de Mondeville H. Spasm and Other Complications. In *The Surgery of Henri de Mondeville. I.* Bloomington, IN: XLibris; 2003, pp. 493–510.
46. de Mondeville H. The Choice of Method of Treatment. In *The Surgery of Henri de Mondeville. I.* Bloomington, IN: XLibris; 2003, p. 299.
47. de Mondeville H. The Conditions which Determine when to renew Dressings. In *The Surgery of Henri de Mondeville 1.* Bloomington, IN: XLibris; 2003, pp. 308–10.
48. de Mondeville H. The Steps to be Taken in Treating different Categories of Wounds by the Modern Method. In *The Surgery of Henri de Mondeville. I.* Bloomington, IN: XLibris; 2003, pp. 329–44.
49. de Mondeville H. The Therapeutic Diminution of Blood Useful and Necessary for the Body, as it should be practiced in individual Cases, according to the Art of Medicine and Surgery. In *The Surgery of Henri de Mondeville 1.* Bloomington, IN: XLibris; 2003, pp. 234–94.
50. de Mondeville H. Fistulas. In *The Surgery of Henri de Mondeville. II.* Bloomington, IN: XLibris; 2003, pp. 625–35.
51. de Mondeville H. Cancerous Ulcers. In *The Surgery of Henri de Mondeville. II.* Bloomington, IN: XLibris; 2003, pp. 636–52.
52. de Mondeville H. Phlebotomy and its Uses. In *The Surgery of Henri de Mondeville. II.* Bloomington, IN: XLibris; 2003, pp. 696–728.
53. de Mondeville H. Lepers and Leprosy. In *The Surgery of Henri de Mondeville. II.* Bloomington, IN: XLibris; 2003, pp. 783–96.
54. de Mondeville H. Aposthems derived from a single non-natural humor or from several of the mixed type, that is, a cancerous aposthem. In *The Surgery of Henri de Mondeville. II.* Bloomington, IN: XLibris; 2003, pp. 877–81.
55. de Mondeville H. Treatment of aposthems of the anterior chest wall. In *The Surgery of Henri de Mondeville. II.* Bloomington, IN: XLibris; 2003, pp. 895–9.
56. de Mondeville H. Ten Principles. In *The Surgery of Henri de Mondeville. 1.* Bloomington, IN: XLibris; 2003, pp. 191–6.
57. de Mondeville H. How To Use Cauteries. In *The Surgery of Henri de Mondeville. II.* Bloomington, IN: XLibris; 2003, pp. 679–85.
58. de Mondeville H. Fifty-two Contingents and particular Conditions in Diseases in Notable XIV. In *The Surgery of Henri de Mondeville. I.* Bloomington, IN: XLibris; 2003, pp. 289–90.

59. de Mondeville H. Surgical Cauterization and its Uses. In *The Surgery of Henri de Mondeville. II*. Bloomington, IN: XLibris; 2003, pp. 674–96.
60. Rosenman LD. Introduction. In *The Surgery of Jehan Yperman*. Bloomington, IN: XLibris; 2003, pp. 21–33.
61. Jones P. Yperman, Jan. In: Bynum WBH, editor. *Dictionary of Medical Biography S - Z*. London: Greenwood Press; 2007, pp. 1340–1.
62. Yperman J. The Treatment of the Tumor of the Head called Testudo.In *The Surgery of Master Jehan Yperman*. Bloomington, IN: XLibris; 2002, pp. 106–7.
63. Yperman J. Head Wounds Inflicted by Sharp Corners of the Blades of Cleavers, Knives or Hatchets, or by the Points of Swords. In *The Surgery of Jehan Yperman*. Bloomington, IN: XLibris; 2003, pp. 67–70.
64. Yperman J. Removal of Thorns and other Projectiles without Incisions. In *The Surgery of Master Jehan Yperman*. Bloomington, IN: XLibris; 2002, pp. 92–3.
65. de Chauliac G. *The Major Surgery of Guy de Chauliac an English Translation*. Bloomington, IN: XLibris Corporation; 2005.
66. de Chauliac G. The Requirements for All Surgeons. In *The Major Surgery of Guy de Chauliac: An English Translation*. Bloomington, IN: XLibris; 2007, pp. 125–7.
67. de Chauliac G. Wounds in General. In *The Major Surgery of Guy de Chauliac an English Translation*. Bloomington, IN: XLibris Corporation; 2007, pp. 273–95.
68. de Chauliac G. Useless Parts, When to Amputate, Dead Limbs, Redundant Digits, Embalming Bodies. In *The Major Surgery of Guy de Chauliac an English Translation*. Bloomington, IN: XLibris Corporation; 2007, pp. 476–9.
69. de Chauliac G. The Mouth. In *The Major Surgery of Guy de Chauliac: An English Translation*. Bloomington, IN: XLibris; 2007, pp. 526–37.
70. de Chauliac G. Cutting for Stone. In *The Major Surgery of Guy de Chauliac: An English Translation*. Bloomington, IN: XLibris; 2007, p. 559.
71. de Chauliac G. Groin Hernias, and Operations. In *The Major Surgery of Guy de Chauliac: An English Translation*. Bloomington, IN: XLibris; 2007, pp. 544–51.
72. de Chauliac G. Within the Eye: Caratacts, Gutta Serena, Defective Vision. In *The Major Surgery of Guy de Chauliac: An English Translation*. Bloomington, IN: XLibris; 2007, pp. 513–20.
73. de Chauliac G. Aposthems, Pustules, and Exitures in General. In *The Major Surgery of Guy de Chauliac: An English Translation*. Bloomington, IN: XLibris; 2007, pp. 177–90.
74. de Chauliac G. Palliation. In *The Major Surgery of Guy de Chauliac: An English Translation*. Bloomington, IN: XLibris; 2007, pp. 371–2.
75. de Chauliac G. Signs of Fistulas. In *The Major Surgery of Guy de Chauliac: An English Translation*. Bloomington, IN: XLibris; 2007, pp. 399–400.
76. de Chauliac G. Cauteries: Indications and definition. In *The Major Surgery of Guy de Chauliac: An English Translation*. Bloomington, IN: XLibris; 2007, pp. 597–602.
77. de Chauliac G. Treatments for Nasal Ulcers and Polyps. In *The Major Surgery of Guy de Chauliac: An English Translation*. Bloomington, IN: XLibris; 2007, pp. 383–4.
78. de Chauliac G. Hemorrhoids at the Anus. In *The Major Surgery of Guy de Chauliac: An English Translation*. Bloomington, IN: XLibris; 2007, pp. 394–8.
79. de Chauliac G. Toothache in General. In *The Major Surgery of Guy de Chauliac: An English Translation*. Bloomington, IN: XLibris; 2007, p. 531.
80. de Chauliac G. Phlebotomy, Cupping, Leeches. In *The Major Surgery of Guy de Chauliac: An English Translation*. Bloomington, IN: XLibris; 2007, pp. 572–88.
81. Byrne JP. *Demographic Effects of Plague: Europe 1347 - 1400 Encyclopedia of the Black Death*. Denver, CO: ABC-CLIO; 2012, pp. 108–9.
82. Ziegler P. *The Black Death*. Rockville, MD: American Heritage Publishing; 2016.

83. Byrne JP. Flagellants. In *Encyclopedia of the Black Death*. Denver, CO: ABC-CLIO; 2012, pp. 143–5.
84. Hecker IFC. *The Black Death in the Fourteenth Century*. London: A. Schloss; 1833.
85. Hultåker Ö. (Ed.) Family and Disaster. *International Journal of Mass Emergencies*. 1983; 1: 7–18.
86. Byrne JP. Abandonment. In *Encyclopedia of the Black Death*. Denver, CO: ABC-CLIO; 2012, p. 1.
87. de Chauliac G. Treatise II The Aposthems. Doctrine II Eight Chapters: Aposthems in Particular Places. In *The Major Surgery of Guy de Chauliac an English Translation*. Bloomington, IN: XLibris Corporation; 2007, pp. 247–50.
88. Cantor NF. Aftermath. In *In the Wake of the Plague*. New York: The Free Press; 2001, pp. 130–42.

5 Changing Anatomy

CLASSICAL TEACHING

Accurate study of anatomy requires familiarity with the body, which can only be acquired by the dissection of corpses. With the exception of a few decades in the first half of the third century BC, dissection had been unacceptable in the classical worlds of Ancient Greece and Rome. In ancient Greece, this was based on the concept that human corpses were unclean and anyone who touched them would subsequently require purification [1]. In ancient Rome, the dissection of dead human bodies was not considered acceptable, so that even Galen did not attempt to undertake it [2]. There was a further dislike of dissection through Islam because of a belief that the body could still feel pain after death [3]. Thus, anatomy was not based on experience of the human body but on the teachings of long-dead authors who based their information on the dissection of animals. While this is understandable, given the social pressures governing human dissection, it is disheartening. Anatomy is the only medical science based exclusively on observation and description. Dissection could have provided surgeons with accurate information on which to base their profession during classical times. In the event, this information would sadly not be available until the sixteenth century.

CHRISTIAN MEDICAL EDUCATION

Following the dismantling of the western Roman Empire, there was no subsequent temporal authority. However, in a changing world, the Catholic Church became increasingly influential, subsequently powerful, and finally wealthy. It was a great landowner. Over time, it came to dominate academic endeavour in the monasteries. As wealth in society increased during the Middle Ages, one of its expressions was the development of towns of increasing size, and many of these towns included cathedrals. (It has been shown that cathedral building correlated with per capita GDP and earnings [4]). One of the consequences of these cathedrals was that they became centres of learning, including medical education, and universities would come to develop from them.

The Church and Dissection

In some quarters of the church, there was a dislike of the dissection of corpses, as shown by St Augustine of Hippo:

> *It pleased the ancient anatomists to examine the viscera of the death to learn in what way they died, but for us humanitas prohibits this [5].*

DOI: 10.1201/9781003748816-5

However, the Christian church did not exercise an outright ban on dissecting the dead, and while a clear picture is not available, examples of dissection started to be recorded. The first of these occurred in 1111 AD. It concerned King Sigurd I Crusader of Norway, and was written up by the historian, William of Malmesbury, in 1125, in his book about the English Kings. This happened because in 1111 King Henry I of England, grandson of William the Conqueror, was on friendly terms with King Sigurd. So, Sigurd stayed in England for the winter before his crusade, which is how the following story came to be included in a book on English kings. It reads as follows:

> *By a change of route he came to Constantinople, and there fixed a ship with golden serpents for its figurehead on the pinnacle of St Sophia as a trophy. In that same city his men began to die like flies, and he himself thought out a remedy, making the survivors drink wine more sparingly, and not unless mixed with water. Such was his penetrating intelligence: he put a pig's liver into the unmixed wine, and finding it soon dissolve away in the harsh liquor, he first foretold that the same thing would happen in the human body, and then obtained visual confirmation by post-mortem examination of one who had died [6].*

The Norwegian king's method of analysis and solution to a question were signs of individual brilliance but was not related to any specific change in the academic milieu. King Sigurd was not interested in academic anatomy studies, but rather he wanted to determine the cause of death. The next dissecting innovators were reported roughly a century later. The eminent medical historian Charles Singer, suggested that William of Saliceto (1210–1277) described the interior of the thorax with such precision that it was probable that he had dissected the region in corpses [7]. Another report of dissection was to be found in the chronicle of a Franciscan monk, Salimbene of Parma, who published in 1286, just a decade after William of Saliceto's death. Salimbene stated that during a pestilence affecting both men and hens, a physician in Cremona had opened several hens to find an abscess at the tip of the heart. A dead man was also opened and found to have the same lesion [5, 8]. All these indicators of burgeoning dissection were concerned with autopsies. Yet earlier in the thirteenth century, in 1231 in southern Italy, Frederick II, King of Naples, and Holy Roman Emperor commanded that a surgeon could only be licensed after five years of studies. It was further decreed that a human body should be dissected at least once every five years for anatomical studies [9].

These events were unsystematic and disseminated, but there now came a major change, in the form of Mondino de Luzzi (1270 to 1326), who was made professor of anatomy in Bologna in 1306. However, before considering Mondino's contributions, it is necessary to examine the anatomical concepts current at his time.

HENRI DE MONDEVILLE'S ANATOMICAL CONCEPTS

Medieval surgeons based their ideas of anatomy on the work of Galen. It would be easy to believe that surgeons so trained would be aware of the relevant structures and their details and would mainly err in terms of their interrelationships and functions.

Nothing could be further from the truth. Henri de Mandeville (1260 to 1316), working in Paris, was only ten years older than Mondino, thus a close contemporary. There is a fairly substantial section on anatomy in his work on surgery. He begins this by defining the extent and limits of anatomical knowledge as follows:

1. *An operating surgeon should know the anatomy.*
2. *What anatomy is.*
3. *The etymology of the word.*
4. *What is a member and how it is divided?*
5. *What we know about all the members together and what they consist of, and the same for the entire body.*

The first four points are clear enough. Point five is less clear, but classification follows with the next heading:

> *The Anatomy of Similar (Consemblable) Parts (Members), Simple and Composite.*

The explanation of this heading is as follows.

A simple consemblable is composed of constituents which are all the same. (This is what we today would call a tissue.) A composite consemblable is composed of various simples in one locality, such as a hand or a finger. (That is what we today would call a part.) However, de Mondeville's notions of a part (member) are rather different from ours. He explains:

> *A Member is a solid part of the body formed at the first coming together of its humors, just as the humors are formed from the first admixture of the aliments, and the aliments are a mixture of their own elements.*

This is a great distance from modern thinking. There are further details. De Mondeville tells us:

> *As to the fifth Proposition in our Introduction, the subdivisions of members, you should know that the similars (i.e. consemblables) are all the elements that join in the function of the member, whether they be simple such as flesh or nerve, or are composite, such as a cord, muscle, hand or finger all of which are part of an arm.*

Finally, there is a further subdivision of parts (members).

> *Some of the Similars (consemblables) are spermatic and some are non-spermatic.*

He goes on to explain what this means.

> *The six purely spermatic consemblable members are bone, cartilage, ligaments, nerves, arteries and veins. The five nonspermatic consemblable members are flesh, fat, fatty panniculus, lard (internal fat) and fiber [10].*

In addition to the strangeness of his anatomical principles, De Mondeville, in his clinical writings, demonstrated a truly worrying lack of accurate anatomical relationships, as shown in the following passage.

> *The woman's breasts are connected to the uterus by veins that bring menstrual blood to them. They digest it and change its color from red to white, which is the color of the mammary flesh. The process is similar to what happens to the white chyle which the stomach delivers to the liver where it is changed to red (i.e. to the blood of nutrition) by digestion in a red organ. Milk is white because it is the product of digestion by white breast tissues, and it is the residue of the nourishment that serves the breast itself. So it is that a structure must be nourished by substances that resemble it [11].*

There was a stark need to change the medieval approach to anatomy.

MONDINO'S CONTRIBUTION

The first step on the road to acquiring accurate knowledge of human anatomy came with the appointment of Mondino de' Luzzi (ca. 1270–1326) to the Chair of Anatomy in Bologna, where he introduced public dissection into the medical curriculum in 1313. It has been assumed that he had the blessing of the Pope since the dissections were undertaken with municipal and ecclesiastical approval. It may, however, be noted that formal approval of dissection did not appear in the university statutes until 1405 [7]. However, these dissections were not a demonstration of the anatomy in front of those present. Instead, Mondino read from the texts of Aristotle, Galen, and Avicenna and the visible structures were indicated with reference to the authoritative texts by the dissector [12, 13]. Despite the weakness of his method, Mondino made a second important contribution. He wrote the first textbook on anatomy, which previously had only been presented as a section in surgical texts [14]. This arrangement is illustrated by Figure 5.1 taken from a printed edition of Mondino's Anatomy text from 1541 [15].

Since Mondino's original Anathomia was a manuscript, it included no anatomical illustrations. However, in the printed edition from which Figure 5.1 was taken, there were also illustrations of anatomy.

ILLUSTRATIONS

The primary purpose of a text on surgery is to inform the student reader of the knowledge and methods of an expert. In this context, accurate illustration is most important. The earliest surgical book with illustrations is the 'Buch der Chirurgie' by the German, Hieronymus Brunschwig. It was published in Strasbourg in 1497 [16]. The illustrations show oversimplified images of injured patients sitting down or lying in bed surrounded by well-sketched observers. They are attractive images, but not really very helpful as aids to instruction (see Figure 5.2). The illustrator was not named. Another book, also published in Strasbourg in 1517, was the 'Feldbuch der Wundarznei' (Field Book of Wound Medicine) by Hans von Gersdorff. It contains

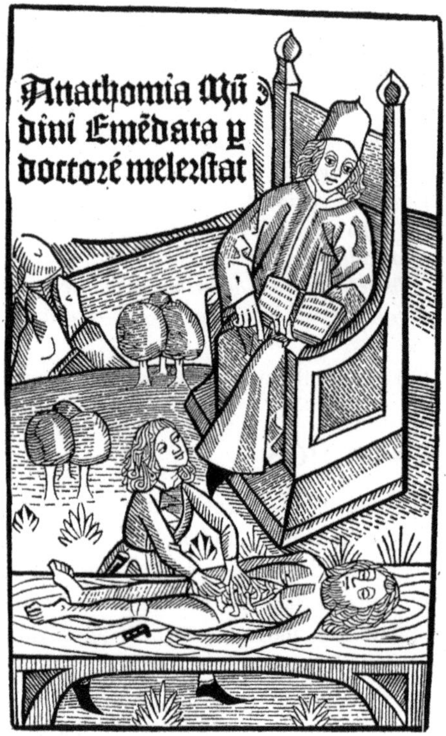

FIGURE 5.1 Mondino supervising dissection.

Mondino introduced the practice of dissection to anatomical teaching. However, he sat at a distance, relaxing, and an assistant did the actual work. Moreover, Mondino's words did not describe what was being demonstrated but rather what was consistent with ancient texts.

much more intricate illustrations attributed to a well-known artist called Hans Wechtlin. Surgical manoeuvres are illustrated, though again they are more dramatic than realistic.

However, there are many illustrations of elegantly contrived mechanical devices designed to facilitate surgical procedures. The quality of the images meant that the book had a great impact (see Figure 5.3). Since these two books were not textbooks of anatomy, there are no anatomical illustrations. On the other hand, they provide evidence of the quality of illustration, which was possible at the time of their publication.

BERENGARIO DA CARPI (1460–1530)

In 1517, Berengario published his book on cranial injuries. This contains no images of people, anatomy, or surgical situations. It includes only images of instruments.

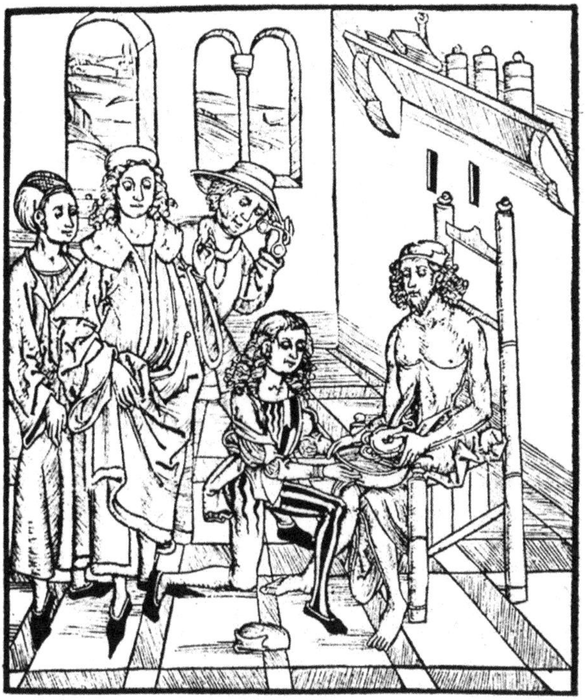

FIGURE 5.2 Illustration from Brunschwig's Buch der Chirurgie.

An illustration from the first surgical textbook with illustrations, published soon after the invention of the printing press. The image includes a lot of social detail, a rather diagrammatic representation of an abdominal injury with extrusion of the gut. But it is not anatomically accurate enough to have been useful to surgeons in training.

However, since the design was revolutionary, the images were important, even if not of the highest quality, as shown in Figure 5.4. The drawing is barely of professional quality, but it does demonstrate the important parts of the new drill, which is for two hands, with a brace and bit design and also can take interchangeable bits. This was a major design improvement.

In 1522, more than two centuries after Mondino, Berengario da Carpi published a book on anatomy, *Isagogae Breves*. It opens with a much more modern-sounding paragraph:

> *But we must begin with the body as a whole, i.e., from the whole as from something that is better known; first, from a cadaver laid supine in a place suitable for cutting and displaying. Before this, the cadaver must be washed, its hair shaven, and well cleaned of dirt from head to feet. You should know that the body is to be divided into four parts: that is, into three prominent cavities and the extremities, that is, hands and feet along with certain other things [17].*

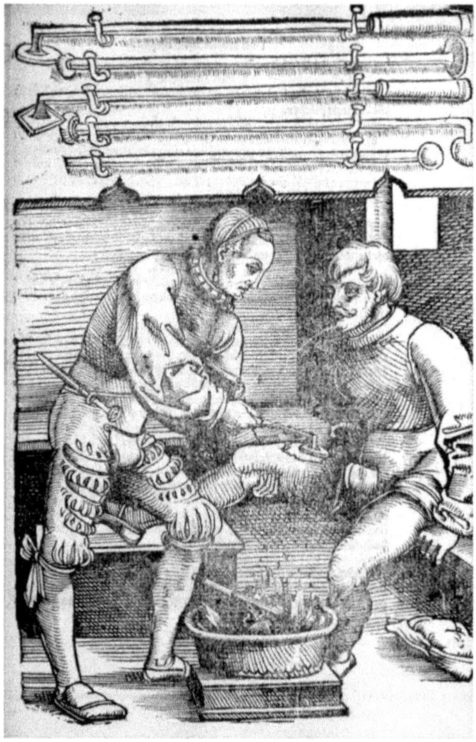

FIGURE 5.3 Image from von Gersdorff's Feldbuch der Wundarznei.

The drawing is much more detailed and realistic than the image from the Brunschwig book. While it is dramatic, it is surgically unrealistic. The patient is sitting calmly while a cautery is stopping bleeding from his thigh. In reality, he would be supine and needing restraint, on account of the pain.

Not only is the terminology more familiar to a modern reader, but also the book is the first text on anatomy to include illustrations. Unfortunately, they are not of such a high quality as those in the German books on surgery. Figure 5.5 shows an image of the human seen from the side. The anatomical proportions are adequate, but it lacks accurate anatomical detail.

VESALIUS (1514 TO 1564)

The application of perspective to woodcuts produced by members of Titian's School of Art was essential in the production of a vital book which would be an important component in the development of scientific medicine. This book was Vesalius' monograph 'De Humani Corporis Fabrica' (On the Fabric of the Human Body) published in 1543.

Every physician learns that modern anatomy began with Vesalius. However, we are not routinely taught about how this came about. Vesalius was born into a distinguished medical family with contacts with royalty and universities. He started his formal education in Louvain in 1528 at the age of fourteen, and his major studies

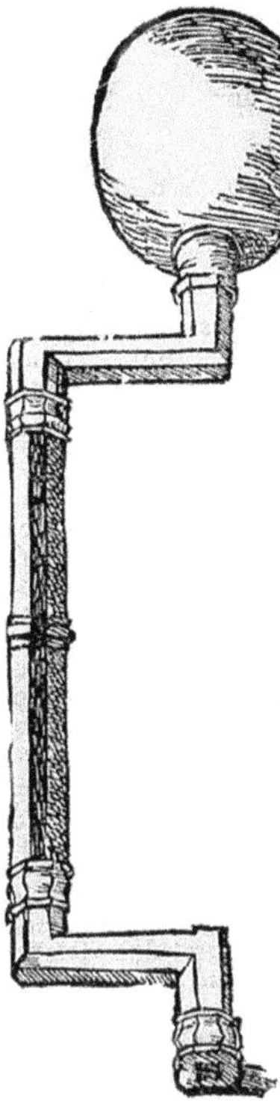

FIGURE 5.4 Berengario's trepan.

While not elegant or detailed, this image nonetheless quite adequately shows an instrument which introduced a new technique for trepanation, making it easier to control.

were the languages of Latin, Greek, and Hebrew. It is recorded that while his Latin was fluent, his Greek was patchy and his Hebrew non-existent [8]. Nonetheless, fluent Latin gave him access to a wide range of knowledge. In 1533, at the age of nineteen, he moved to Paris to begin his formal medical education. Paris was prestigious but conservative, and dissection, which had become legal, was only rarely practiced. Medical knowledge came from Arabic sources and from Arabic translations of the ancient masters. However, this was the time of the appearance of new translations of Galen directly into Latin, which meant that a better quality of writing became thereby available. It is widely believed that Vesalius was opposed to Galen's teachings, but this is not the case. Rather, he refused to accept them slavishly as gospel and rather tested them against the results of observation and noted discrepancies. While there was little dissection in Paris in his three years there, he increasingly took part in the presentation of dissections. In the tradition initiated 200 years earlier in Bologna by Mondino and continued in the same place at the beginning of the sixteenth century by Giacomo Berengario da Carpi, he performed his own dissections and based his writings on what he observed personally.

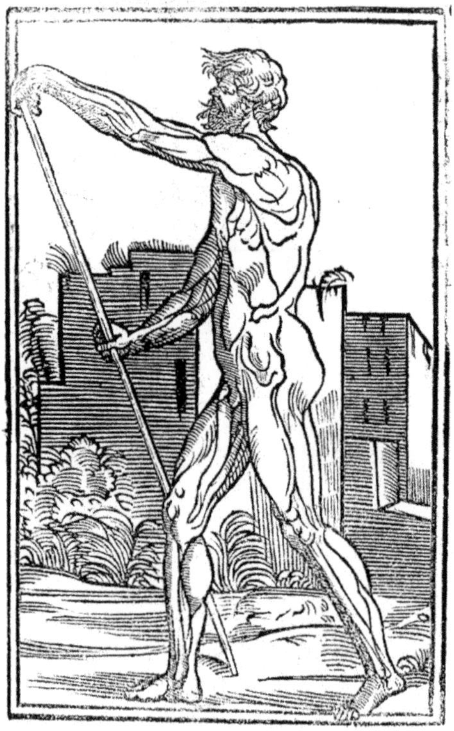

FIGURE 5.5 Illustration from Berengario's Isagogae Breves

The anatomical proportions are adequate, but it is not clear to what extent the skin has been removed, and the muscles shown are not anatomically accurate.

Vesalius and his colleagues visited the Gibbet of Montfaucon, where executed bodies were brought to rot to a condition that facilitated disposal. It was haunted by crows and savage dogs, but was a rich source of material for avid anatomists. There was also the Cemetery of the Innocents, whence, as Vesalius remarked, there was "*an abundant supply when I first studied the bone*" [18]. This is so incredibly far removed from the conditions of study in a modern medical school, where the corpses used for dissection are contained within clean, carefully maintained systems of storage.

Vesalius moved back to Louvain because of the war and, in 1537, completed his baccalaureate. By December of that year, he had moved to Padua, where he was examined for the degree of Doctor of Medicine, which he obtained with the highest distinction. The following day, he was appointed professor of surgery in Padua at the tender age of twenty-three [18].

This was an appointment which required the teaching of anatomy. He was well-liked and influential because he did not delegate dissection to others but undertook it himself. This was novel and popular, and his classes were crowded. Moreover, he wrote down and published his anatomical findings with elegant illustrations because printing was available and because he had access to first-rate artists trained in the laws of perspective (see Figure 5.6). He found that his students welcomed these illustrations, and in 1538 he published six large plates called the Tabulae Sex illustrating the skeleton from front, back, and side together with the veins, arteries, and liver in a way to illustrate the physiology of Galen [19]. It may be mentioned that he dissected the brain in situ, taking horizontal sections from above downwards. It could take six heads to produce brain illustrations because the brains decomposed so quickly [18].

Vesalius remained a thorough student of Galen and contributed to the publication of the old master's works in Latin in 1541. If nothing else, this is evidence that Vesalius did not oppose all of Galen's teachings. Nonetheless, like Berengario Da Carpi, he was willing to believe the evidence of his own eyes rather than the teachings of the past. Vesalius is credited with much-improved illustrations of the brain, but he described two anatomically important errors, one concerning the arterial supply to the brain and the other concerning the classification of the cranial nerves. In his Tabulae, published in 1538, he perpetuated the error that arterial blood reached the brain via a marvellous network or rete mirabile, which is not present in humans.

It should be remembered that Berengario Da Carpi had denied the presence of this rete mirabilis in his anatomy book 'Isagogae Breves,' published fifteen years before Vesalius' 'Tabulae.' Five years later, in the Fabrica, Vesalius had corrected this error [20, 21]. Thus, he was learning from observation as time passed. Vesalius also described seven cranial nerves, which look similar to the descriptions in Galen's 'On Anatomical Procedures' [22]. Thomas Willis (1621 to 1675) would come closer to an accurate description of the cranial nerves in his book 'Cerebri Anatome' published in 1664 [23]. The final modern description came from Samuel Thomas Soemmerring (1755–1830) in 1778 [24]. However, none of these gentlemen was surgeons concerned with the pain of operating.

AMBROISE PARÉ (1510 TO 1590)

It was finally in Ambroise Paré's monumental surgical text that anatomical illustrations of the highest quality were married to a text on surgery. In the French original, the illustrations are stated to be by Vesalius [25]. It would seem that Paré was well aware of Vesalius. He wrote:

> *The figures of Anatomy: most of which I have borrowed from Andre Vesal, a rare man, & the first of his time in this era of Medicine [25].*

Figure 5.6 in the English edition of Paré's text bears the legend 'the seventh figure of the lower belly'. It is, in fact, a component of plate fifty-eight of Vesalius' Fabrica. It shows just how advanced the images in Paré's book were. They are valuable and accurate images of anatomy, in the age after Vesalius' revolution in the study of the subject.

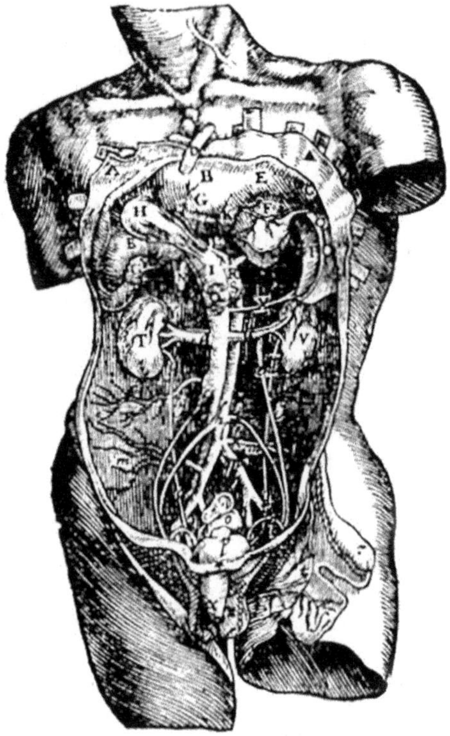

FIGURE 5.6 Abdominal anatomy from the English translation of Paré's surgery textbook.

The image was borrowed by Paré from Plate58 of Vesalius' Fabrica with the permission of the latter. It is an accurate and detailed illustration of the abdominal contents following removal of the intestines. This sort of accurate anatomy provided a basis for significant improvements in surgical technique.

CONCLUSION

The content of this chapter describes how human curiosity battled with ignorance to achieve truth, at least with respect to the structure of the body.

With regard to pain management, it is not possible to be certain that the acquisition of knowledge described in this chapter affected the relationship between surgeon and patient. Nonetheless, from the time of Berengario onwards, descriptions of modifying surgical technique to minimize pain became more or less routine, which was a new development.

REFERENCES

1. von Staden H. The Discovery of the Body: Human Dissection and Its Cultural Contexts in Ancient Greece. *The Yale Journal of Biology and Medicine*. 1992; 6: 223–41.
2. Nutton V. Galenic Medicine. In *Ancient Medicine*. 2nd ed. London and New York: Routledge; 2013, pp. 236–53.

3. Conrad LI. The Arab-Islamic Medical Tradition. In *The Western Medical Tradition.* Cambridge, MA: Cambridge University Press; 2009, pp. 93–138.
4. Buringh E, Campbell BMS, Rijpmaa A, van Zandena JL. Church building and the economy during Europe's 'Age of the Cathedrals', 700–1500 CE. *Explorations in Economic History.* 2020; 76, article ID: 101316.
5. van den Tweel JG, Taylor CR. The rise and fall of the autopsy. *Virchows Archiv.* 2013; 462: 371–80.
6. Mynors RAB, Thomson RM, Winterbottom M (Eds.). *William of Malmesbury: Gesta Regum Anglorum, The History of the English Kings 1.* Oxford: Clarendon Press; 1998, pp. 742–3.
7. Singer C. The Middle Ages and Renaissance 1050 - 1543. In *A Short History of Anatomy from the Greeks to Harvey.* New York: Dover Publications Inc; 1972, pp. 66–110.
8. O'Malley CD. Pre Vesalian Anatomy. In *Andreas Vesalius of Brussels 1514 - 1564.* Berkeley, CA: University of California Press; 1964, pp. 9–40.
9. Ghosh SK. Human Cadaveric Dissection: A Historical Account from Ancient Greece to the Modern Era. *Anatomy and Cell Biology.* 2015; 48(3): 153–69.
10. de Mondeville H. The Anatomy of Similar (Consemblable) Parts (Members), Simple and Composite. In *The Surgery of Henri de Mondeville. 1.* Bloomington, IN: XLibris; 2003, pp. 117–9.
11. de Mondeville H. The Chest and its Contents. In *The Surgery of Henri de Mondeville. 1.* Bloomington, IN: XLibris; 2003, pp. 154–5.
12. Standring S. A Brief History of Topographical Anatomy. *Journal of Anatomy.* 2016; 229: 33–62.
13. Infusino MH, Win D, O'Neill YV. Mondino's Book and the Human Body. *Vesalius.* 1995; 1: 71–6.
14. Malomo AO, Idown OE, Osuagwu FC. Lessons from History: Human Anatomy, from the Origin to the Renaissance. *International Journal of Morphology.* 2006; 24(1): 99–104.
15. Luzzi Md. *Anatomia.* Marburg: Christian Egenolphi; 1541.
16. Bruschwig H. *Buch der Cirurgie.* Strasbourg: Johann Grüninger; 1497.
17. Da Carpi B. *Isagogae Breves.* Chicago: University of Chicago Press; 1959.
18. Catani M, Sandrone S. Dissecting the Fabrica. In *Brain Renaissance from Vesalius to Modern Neuroscience.* Oxford: Oxford University Press; 2015, pp. 23–7.
19. Saunders JBdM, O'Malley CD. The Plates from the Tabulae Sex. In *The Anatomical Drawings of Andreas Vesalius.* New York: Crown Publishers; 1982, pp. 233–47.
20. Russell GA. Vesalius and the Emergence of Veridical Representation in Renaissance Anatomy. *Progress in Brain Research.* 2013; 2013: 3–32.
21. Clarke E, Dewhurst K. *Transition: The Rete Mirabile. An Illustrated History of Brain Function.* Oxford: Sandford Publications; 1972, pp. 56–9.
22. Galen. The Cranial Nerves. In: Lyons MC, Towers B, editors. *Galen on Anatomical Procedures, The Later Books.* Cambridge, MA: Cambridge University Press; 2010, pp. 8–10.
23. Arráez-Aybar L-A, Alvarez P, Fuentes-Redondo T, Bueno-Lopéz JL. Thomas Willis, a Pioneer in Translational Research in Anatomy [on the 350th anniversary of Cerebri Anatome]. *Journal of Anatomy.* 2015; 226: 289–300.
24. Pearce JMS. The Naming of Cranial Nerves. *European Neurology* 2017; 77: 303–6.
25. Park MT, Mignucci-Jiménez G, Houlihan LM. Management of Injuries on the 16th-Century Battlefield: Ambroise Paré's Contributions to Neurosurgery and Functional Recovery. *Neurosurgical Focus.* 2022; 53(3): 1–12.

6 Surgical Pain – Renaissance

INTRODUCTION

The surgeons assessed in this chapter lived in a different milieu from those described in earlier chapters, and important differences were unavoidable. The printing press made medical manuscripts easily available. In particular, Celsus' 'De Medicina' had been rediscovered by Pope Nicholas V in 1443 [1]. It was the first medical text published with the new printing press, and it became an influential part of the medical curriculum. It may be mentioned that the book was published when Berengario was eighteen years old. He was the first of the surgeons mentioned so far in this book to have access to Celsus' seminal work, and he mentioned him multiple times.

The profession of surgery was changing. None of the surgeons mentioned in this chapter were ordained priest. Three of them, Berengario da Carpi, Ambroise Paré, and John Woodall, were what were called barber surgeons with a social standing inferior to academic surgeons. They were not allowed to prescribe medicines, and major operations could only be undertaken in the presence of a physician [2]. Berengario's text was written in Latin, but the works of Paré, Lowe, and Woodall were all in the vernacular. Lowe had enough Latin for parts of the introduction of his book, but there is no evidence that either Paré or Woodall had learned the language. Finally, the personal interactions based on social rank, called feudalism, were in decline [3].

GIACOMO BERENGARIO DA CARPI (1460 TO 1530)

Berengario was a formidable surgeon and the son of a barber-surgeon, a sign of the changing times. He was also an anatomist and correctly observed errors in the teachings of Galen, which nonetheless continued to be accepted for many years. Although he studied and later taught at the Bologna medical school, he had poor Latin, which could have hindered the dissemination of his work. He acquired the rank of Master of Arts and Medicine on 3 August 1489 at the age of twenty-nine. Interestingly, the roll recording his success had the note:

> "*hic evasit magnum anatomicum*" ('…this was the beginning of a great anatomist') [4].

This was a prescient comment indeed. Da Carpi is an example of a man without the formally acceptable education of the clergy, yet who was much sought after by even the most exalted persons in the land, an example of the regression of feudalism. His text 'De Fractura Cranii' was published in 1518 [5]. This was the first book ever

DOI: 10.1201/9781003748816-6

published to be concerned solely with a neurosurgical topic. In the present context, it is the only text that is limited to cranial injury.

Pain of Surgery

Berengario, like his medieval predecessors, noted that patients were scared of cranial surgery. He made the following statement to guide surgeons performing trepanation.

> *When this operation is completed the wound should be filled with tow from which tents are made without heat which are the same as those soaked in egg white and placed in the wound in cases where a great flow of blood is not to be feared. I take the white of an entire egg beaten with a moderate amount of rose oil because it soothes the pain better. It should be left in place for one day until the tent is well dried out because when the lips of the wound are more dry they remain more open and the physician can operate better on the open rather than the closed wound and with less pain to the patient. Physicians should always observe this procedure when they intend to perform trepanation or another operation because when the lips are well opened contact with the instruments and thus damage on the lips is avoided. This contact causes pain which is difficult for the patient to bear nor can he endure such operations because he is forced to suffer more and pain may cause his death [6].*

Thus, Berengario took care to minimize the pain of surgery during trepanation by making sure to keep the skin opening edges away from the surgical instruments. (Trepanation is the operation where some skull bone is penetrated, usually with a circular saw. It is done to access the contents of the skull when injury or other cause for concern is suspected.) In addition, in the event of a possible pericranial injury, the membrane may be separated from the bone. Berengario specified that although the pericranium is normally pain sensitive, contusion could reduce this sensitivity, facilitating separation of the membrane from the bone. (The pericranium is the membrane that covers and nourishes the exterior of the bones of the skull.) In both these instances, he is adapting the technique to minimize the pain of surgery. Lanfranc had urged gentleness in fracture management as a principle. This protection of skin edges is the first mention of adapting a detail of surgical technique to reduce pain during a specific surgical procedure.

Berengario also paid attention to the mood of the patient, considering it important:

> *the patient should be advised to avoid anger and hate no less than fear, sadness, and fury and to drive out completely from himself every worry because these emotions set the humors in motion and cause bad accidents or concomitants. Rather, he should rejoice as much as he can and be happy; let him seek gaiety, every kind of delight and joy of spirit, but he should shun, however, jokes, song, and everything adapted for setting the humors into motion [7].*

It is well documented that Berengario's behaviour could be objectionable with respect to colleagues [8]. Nonetheless, his writing about the surgery of the cranium expresses more kindness and consideration for patients than any previous author, except perhaps Theodoric (see Chapter 4).

The Pain of Cautery

Cautery and cauterization have four mentions in the text. These merely note the existence of the technique without any comment on its value or use, which might be expected since the text is limited to a consideration of cranial surgery alone.

Analgesics

Berengario is quite clear on the subject of these substances stating:

> *Avoid the juice of poppy and mandragora for they cool the patient and harm him [6].*

The traditional dislike of analgesics is maintained.

Phlebotomy

There is no comment on the technique of phlebotomy and its possible complications.

AMBROISE PARÉ (1510 TO 1590)

The name of Ambroise Paré is familiar to most, if not all, engaged in the practice of surgery. He was of humble origins and qualified eventually as a Master Barber-Surgeon. Nonetheless, during his education, he spent some time in the famous Hôtel Dieu hospital in Paris. Despite his humble origins, he ended up as surgeon to four successive French kings. His gentleness and clinical skill were greatly regarded [9].

Little is known of Ambroise Paré's background. He was born in Laval, a town south-west of Paris. He never mastered Latin and Greek and thus could not become an academic surgeon [10]. Despite this, he also became the prime surgeon of his time. Paré's textbook on surgery was first published in 1564. He had definite ideas about the pain inflicted by the surgeon's knife.

Pain of Surgery

Paré's attitude to pain is a world away from that of his medieval predecessors. Nowhere in his book is there a suggestion that the patient should obey the surgeon and should not question him. At the beginning of his textbook on surgery, Paré paraphrases the wise words of Celsus on the necessary characteristics of surgeons whose work would inevitably inflict pain. He wrote:

> *For my part, I very well like that saying of Celsus: A Chirurgeon must have a strong, stable, and intrepid hand, and a mind resolute and merciless; so that to heal him he taketh in hand, he be not moved to make more haste than the thing requires; or to cut less than is needful; but which doth all things as if he were nothing affected with their cries; not giving heed to the judgement of the vain common people, who speak ill of Chirurgeons because of their ignorance [11].*

Paré also mentions a number of details of technique aimed at reducing the pain of operations. He emphasizes that when suturing a wound, the technique should be adjusted to minimize pain. The parameters that concerned him were the thickness of tissue taken and the apposition of the margins, which should be close but not tightly apposed, so that pus forming under the skin would have a passage for escape [12].

He was also aware of the effect of psychological factors on pain writing:

> *...the mind diverted from the actual cause of pain, is less troubled, or sensible of it [13].*

In another context, he discusses examining patients who had a bullet retained after being shot. Paré had comments on how to find such bullets. Firstly, fingers should be preferred to probes, because probes are painful. However, if probes were required, only blunt-ended probes should be used, as they are less painful than those with sharp ends [14]. Once again, he emphasizes minimizing the pain of treatment.

Paré's concern about pain is also reflected in the comment that touching a region of gangrene (See Chapter 2) may be experienced as painful, but this is more due to anxiety than actual pain, since gangrenous tissue has no sensibility [15]. He adjures surgeons to dissect soft tissues, including membranes from the bone, to be amputated before applying the saw, since sawing soft tissue produces severe, avoidable pain [16]. In addition, Paré introduced the notion that using a tourniquet to apply pressure to the limb to be amputated made that limb less sensitive and thereby reduced the pain [17].

He also has comments on pain with respect to inserting a seton. Setons were used in the treatment of a number of conditions, including perianal fistulae. Setons could also be used as a form of counterirritation therapy, where causing a controlled irritation or wound was thought to redirect or reduce symptoms of disease elsewhere, such as chronic headaches and epilepsy. This is shown in Figure 6.1 derived from Scultetus' 'The Chyrurgeons Store-House' [18]. Paré described how he had once used the cautery to incise the skin for the openings through which the thread should be passed. Yet, subsequently, he used the knife and recommended this method to his students because it was less painful. This is another example of changing technique to reduce a patient's discomfort.

Pain of Cautery

The papal surgeon Giovanni de Vigo (1450 to 1535) had written a textbook of surgery. This book taught that gunshot wounds were poisoned and required cauterization with the scalding hot oil of Elders mixed with a little treacle. It is well known that on an occasion in the middle of a battle, when no oil was available, Paré replaced the cauterization with the standard treatment of unpoisoned wounds with a digestive of egg yolk, oil of roses, and turpentine. He suffered a largely sleepless night worrying about the incomplete treatment, but discovered the next day that the patients who had been treated with a digestive were improving much better than those who had been cauterized [19].

What is less familiar is that Paré, at the beginning of his career as a military surgeon and aware of his inexperience, wrote:

> *Now I had read in John de Vigo that wounds made by Gunshot were venenate or poisoned; and that by reason of the Gunpowder; Wherefore for their cure it was expedient*

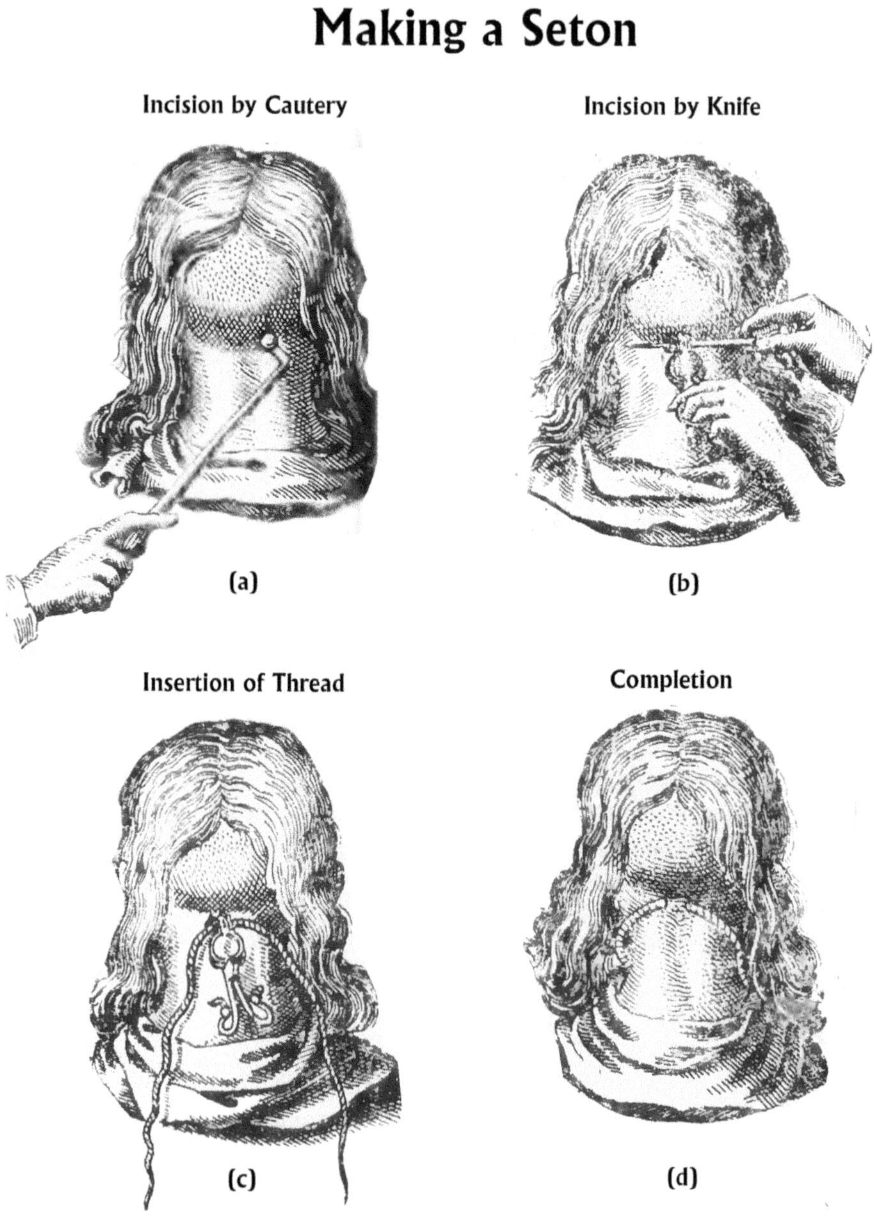

FIGURE 6.1 Insertion of a seton (see text).

Figure 6.1 shows the stages of the procedure. Two small incisions are made in the nape of the neck, either with a cautery or with a scalpel. The coiled thread that constitutes the seton is then passed through the two incisions and finally left in situ. It was believed that such an arrangement would cause chronic irritation, which would counteract chronic headaches or epilepsy.

to burn or cauterize them with oil of Elders scalding hot, with a little Treacle mixed therewith. But for that I gave no great credit neither to the author, nor remedy because I knew that caustics could not be powred into wounds., without excessive pain; I, before would run a hazard., determined to see whether the Chirurgeons, who went with me in the army, used any other manner of dressing to these wounds. I observed and saw that all of them used that Method of dressing which Vigo prescribes; and that they filled as full as they could,-the wounds made by Gunshot with Tents and pledgets dipped in this scalding Oil, at the first dressings; which encouraged me to do the like to those, who came to be dressed of me [19].

He was thus already open for change when the accident produced by absent oil occurred and he was more than ready to change his practice to reduce pain. This is yet another example of changing treatment to reduce pain and also of an attitude that indicated preventing pain was a priority with him.

Paré describes how actual cautery instruments are multiple to manage the varying locations and extents of lesions to be burned. However, he noted that patients are terrified of actual cautery in which situation potential cautery was to be preferred [20].

Principles of Pain Management during Operations

It may be seen from the examination of the writings of Paré outlined above that to a greater degree than any predecessor, he exercised himself to adjust his surgical technique to minimize the suffering of the patient, while motivated by Celsus' principle of ensuring that an operation was as adequate as it could be.

Analgesics

There is no mention of analgesic medication to reduce the pain of surgery.

Phlebotomy

There had been intermittent comments on the risks associated with damage to nerves or tendons during phlebotomy. There had never been any mention of useful treatment. Paré was the first to mention that while phlebotomy could be complicated by intense pain if an adjacent nerve were pricked, it could be treated. He experienced this complication with no less a patient than King Charles IX. For the agonizing pain about which His Majesty complained, Paré applied a variety of plasters that relieved the pain. This was the first mention of treating the pain associated with phlebotomy [21].

PETER LOWE (1550 TO 1610)

Peter Lowe, a younger colleague, also wrote of the qualities required by a surgeon, again demonstrating a debt to Celsus.

There are divers, and first of all as Celsus sayth, that hee bee learned chiefly in those things that appertaine to his art, that he be of a reasonable age, that he have a good hand, as perfit in the left as the right, that hee bee ingenious, subtil, wise, that he tremble not doing his operations, that he have a good eye, that he have good experience in this art, before he begin to practise the same. Also that he has seen and observed of a long time, of learned Chirurgians that he be well mannered, affable, hardy in things certaine, fearfull in thinges doubtfull and dangerous, discrete in judgement of sicknesses, chast, sober, pitifull, that he take his reward according to his cure and the habilitie of the sicke, not regarding avarice [22].

Lowe's practice with gunshot wounds was the same as Paré's, though his justification is the effectiveness of the treatment rather than the avoidance of pain. Indeed, his attitudes are notably similar to those of the medieval surgeons rather than those of Berengario and Paré. When asked.

What conditions ought the sicke to have?

he answers:

Divers also, and first hee must have a good opinion of the Chirurgian that he haue a good hope to be cured of him & be obedient to his counsels, for that availeth much in healing of maladies, that he indure patientlye, that which is done for the recouerie of his health.

Pain of Surgery

There is no mention of the pain of surgery nor of its management.

Pain of Cautery

There is no mention of the pain of cautery as such, but there is a unique description of a detail of technique, the purpose of which must have been to limit pain. Lowe wrote:

First marke the place with thy finger or spot of incke, next make a little emplaister, having a little hole in the middest, either broad or long, as ye shall thinke good, put on the emplaister in such sort, that the marke of the incke appeare through the hole, and then apply the canter [23].

Analgesics

There is no discussion of the use of analgesics to reduce the pain of surgery.

Phlebotomy

There is a detailed description of how to perform a phlebotomy, but there is no accompanying account of complications. Specifically, there is no mention of pain following phlebotomy due to nerve injury [24]. However, there is a description elsewhere of injuries to nerves where it is specified that partial injuries can be more serious and painful than total transection [25].

Summary of Lowe's Approach

The management of pain is always going to be concerned with the character and behaviour of the surgeon and his patient. In the case of Lowe, his behaviour is less patient-orientated and more concerned with professional dignity. This also affected other aspects of his life than patient management. This manifested itself in several different ways. There was no proper institution for medical training in the Scotland of his youth, so he travelled to Paris, where he was educated. Moreover, there is evidence of the importance of prestigious titles to him since he claimed to be a Doctor of the Faculty of Surgery in Paris at the time when there was no such faculty. Moreover, the community of surgeons granted surgeons the title of Master, not Doctor [26, 27]. In addition, he expressed contempt for barber surgeons and the Royal College of Physicians and Surgeons in Glasgow, which Lowe founded excluded barber surgeons, the only surgical college in the British Isles to do so [28]. Lowe was a surgeon of the 'Long Robe', an approved university graduate accepted in the upper classes. This may underlie his rather anachronistic attitude to patients.

JOHN WOODALL (1573 TO 1643)

John Woodall came from a land-owning family in the English Midlands. Little, if anything, is known of his childhood and early education [2]. He began his career in the army and spent several years in Europe, including eight years in Germany and subsequently in the Netherlands and other European countries. He was proficient in German. He was active in the Barber-Surgeons' guild in London and achieved high office. He was also active with the East-India Company as well as other colonial companies. He was commercially successful. His association with a great trading company provided the background for his book on the suitable contents of the chest that accompanied surgeons on their voyages. This book was published in two editions, one in 1617 [29] and one in 1639 [30].

The Pains of Treatment

Woodall's book was an important practical guide for surgeons who would have to work in unstable conditions, with poor lighting and little space. It is this aspect of surgery on which the author concentrates. He has but a little to say about the pain associated with interventions. Nonetheless, he mentions that, like Paré, probing can be painful. He advises that the use of probes should be as limited as possible. Secondly, he notes that while cautery has a place in the treatment of haemorrhage and epilepsy, it has become less popular because of the terror it induces in the patient.

Phlebotomy

There is no mention of the techniques and possible complications of phlebotomy.

CONCLUSION

The four books considered in this chapter had different purposes. Berengario's book concerned skull injuries alone. It outlines details of anatomy and their relevance to management. It also discusses the instruments and techniques involved in opening the cranium. Paré's book is a mammoth account of the nature of diseases, surgical anatomy, principles of treatment, and details of technique. Peter Lowe's book has a similar aim but is much less detailed. John Woodall was primarily concerned with the instruments a naval surgeon should keep available when on board ship.

In this period, excellence in surgery is no longer the monopoly of men with an impressive university education, including familiarity with the Latin language. The most distinguished practitioners, for example, Berengario, had poor Latin, and Paré had none, yet they were the leading surgeons of their time. In addition, both of them included in their texts advice on how to minimize the pain which surgical management must inevitably cause. An exception to this humane trend was provided by Peter Lowe, who, while professionally eminent and politically astute, scorned the barber surgeons and adopted an authoritative attitude to patient management. Even so, the general trend for the period was in the direction of greater respect and sympathy for the patient.

REFERENCES

1. Spivack BS. A.C. Celsus: Roman Medicus. *Journal of the History of Medicine and Allied Sciences*. 1991; 46: 143–57.
2. Appleby JH. Woodall, John (1570 - 1643). In *Oxford Dictionary of National Biography*. Oxford: Oxford University Press; 2008.
3. Cartwright M. *Feudalism 2018*. Available from: https://www.worldhistory.org/Feudalism
4. De Santo NG, Bisaccia C, De Santo LS, De Santo RM, Di Leo VA, Papalia T, et al. Berengario da Carpi. *The American Journal of Nephrology*. 1999; 19: 199–212.
5. Di Ieva A, Gaetani P, Matula C, Sherif C, Skopec M, Tschabitscher M. Berengario da Carpi: A pioneer in neurotraumatology. *Journal of Neurosurgery*. 2011; 114: 1461–70.
6. Carpi BD. Care of External Lesions of the Head. In *Berengario da Carpi on Fracture of the Skull or Cranium Translated into English*. Philadelphia, PA: The American Philosophical Society; 1990, pp. 55–67.
7. Berengario Da Carpi G. Regimen of the Emotions. In *Berengario da Carpi on Fracture of the Skull or Cranium Translated into English*. Philadelphia, PA: The American Philosophical Society; 1990, pp. 83–5.
8. O'Malley CD. *Berengario Da Carpi Giacomo 2008*. Available from: http://www.encyclopedia.com
9. O'Neill YV. Paré, Ambroise. In: Bynum WF, Bynum H, editors. *Dictionay of Medical Biography. 4 (M-R)*. London: Greenwood Press; 2007, pp. 969–73.
10. Packard FR. Birthplace and Lineal Background. In *Life and Times of Ambroise Pare*. New York: Paul B. Hoeber; 1921, pp. 10–26.
11. Johnson T. An Introduction or Compendious Way to Chirurgery: Of Chirurgical Operations. In *The Workes of the Famous Chirurgion Ambroise Pare: Translated out of the Latine and Compared with the French*. London: Richard Cotes; 1649, pp. 1–2.
12. Johnson T. Of Wounds in Generall. In *The Workes of the Famous Chirurgion Ambroise Pare: Translated out of the Latine and Compared with the French*. London: Richard Cotes; 1649, pp. 252–5.

13. Johnson T. Of the Generall Causes of Tumors. In *The Workes of the Famous Chirurgion Ambroise Pare: Translated out of the Latine and Compared with the French.* London: Richard Cotes; 1649, p. 196.
14. Johnson T. A Description of Fit Instruments to Draw Forth Bullets and Other Strange Bodies. In *The Workes of the Famous Chirurgion Ambroise Pare: Translated out of the Latine and Compared with the French.* London: Richard Cotes; 1649, pp. 316–8.
15. Johnson T. The Signs of a Perfect Necrosis or Mortification. In *The Workes of the Famous Chirurgion Ambroise Pare: Translated out of the Latine and Compared with the French.* London: Richard Cotes; 1649, p. 338.
16. Johnson T. How the Section or Amputation Must be Performed. In *The Workes of the Famous Chirurgion Ambroise Pare: Translated out of the Latine and Compared with the French.* London: Richard Cotes; 1649, p. 339.
17. Johnson T. Of the Uses for Which Ligatures Serve. In *The Workes of the Famous Chirurgion Ambroise Pare: Translated out of the Latine and Compared with the French.* London: Richard Cotes; 1649, p. 360.
18. Scultetus J. *The Chyrurgeons Store-House.* London: John Starkey; 1674.
19. Johnson T. The First Discourse Wherein Wounds made by Gunshot are Freed from Being Burnt, or Cauterized According to Vigoes Method. In *The Workes of the Famous Chirurgion Ambroise Pare: Translated out of the Latine and Compared with the French.* London: Richard Cotes; 1649, pp. 309–11.
20. Johnson T. Rules of Surgerie by the Autor. In *The Workes of the Famous Chirurgion Ambroise Pare: Translated Out of the Latine and Compared with the French.* London: Richard Cotes; 1649, p. 752.
21. Johnson T. Of the Cure of the Wounds of the Nervous Parts. In *The Workes of the Famous Chirurgion Ambroise Pare: Translated out of the Latine and Compared with the French.* London: Richard Cotes; 1649, pp. 304–5.
22. Lowe P. The Second Chapter of Chirurgerie in General of Operations and the Instruments of Chirurgerie. In *The Whole Course of Chirurgerie.* London: Thomas Purfoot; 1612.
23. Lowe P. Eigth Treatise of Divers Operations Chirurgicall. Fifth Chapter, of Canters Actual and Potentiall. In *The Whole Course of Chirurgerie.* London: Thomas Purfoot; 1612.
24. Lowe P. Eigth Treatise Of divers operations Chirurgicall, Chapter 1 Of Bleeding and Things Therein to be Observed. In *The Whole Course of Chirurgerie.* London: Thomas Purfoot; 1612.
25. Lowe P. The Sixth Treatise of Woundes. The Seventh Chapter, of Woundes in the Nerues. In *The Whole Course of Chirurgerie.* London: Thomas Purfoot; 1612.
26. Finlayson J. *Account of the Life and Works of Maister Peter Lowe.* Glasgow: James Maclehose & Sons; 1889.
27. Hamilton D. The Troubled Years: 17th Century. In *The Healers: A History of Medicine in Scotland.* Gretna: Firebird Press; 1981.
28. Buchanan WW, Gately JF. Maister Peter Lowe (circa 1550 - 1610): Founder of the Royal College of Physicians Nd Surgeons of Glasgow. *Royal College of Physicians of Edinburgh.* 1999; 29: 338–48.
29. Woodall J. *The Surgeon's Mate or A Treatise Discovering Faithfully and Plainely the Due Contents of the Surgions Chest.* London: Laurence Lisle; 1617.
30. Woodall J. *The Surgeon's Mate or Military and Domestic Surgery.* London: Nicholas Bourne; 1639.

7 Surgical Pain – The Enlightenment

INTRODUCTION

The Enlightenment developed the new intellectual approaches of the Renaissance, in which dogma was questioned and personal observations replaced accepted beliefs. These changes affected surgeons as much as any other group. The dates of the Enlightenment are obviously not precisely delimited, but roughly speaking, it lasted from the end of the Renaissance (1650) to the French Revolution (1789) or maybe a little later. One consequence of this new intellectual approach was that the corpus of agreed knowledge and understanding was continually expanding. Another change is that from this time on, there is more available biographical information concerning the surgeons whose writings are examined. This biographical information includes accounts of the relationships between surgeons and patients, which inevitably have an impact on the management of patients' pain. The first of the great Enlightenment surgeons was an Englishman who played a prominent role in the British Civil War on the side of the King.

RICHARD WISEMAN (1620 TO 1676)

There is a church register record at St. Andrew Undershaft in London of the christening of a Richard Wiseman on 31 December 1620. He was apprenticed to a surgeon named Richard Smith in 1637 at the usual age of sixteen [1]. The apprenticeship ended in 1644, two years after the start of the English Civil War. He joined the Royalists and accompanied them on his wanderings, ending up in 1651 at the final battle of the war at Worcester, where he was captured. While imprisoned in Chester, he was allowed to treat patients, and on moving to London, he obtained the freedom of the Barber-Surgeons' company and was permitted to continue in practice [2]. Following the restoration of his master Charles II in 1660, he was appointed Surgeon to the Person only ten days after Charles' arrival back in England [1]. Towards the end of his life, he published a text called '*Severall Chirurgicall Treatises*'. It was a book with great influence, being republished in many editions [1, 3]. It may also be mentioned that while Wiseman was a barber surgeon and did not possess a university degree, he was nonetheless well informed of the classical teachings of Hippocrates, Celsus, and Galen [3]. He was also familiar with the more modern writings of Falloppius, Guy de Chauliac, and Ambroise Paré. Thus, despite the lack of a formal university education, he was by any measure professionally very well informed.

In addition to his familiarity with classical and recent past teachings, he was up to date, being familiar with Harvey's description of the circulation of the blood. There is evidence for this in the following statement:

 DOI: 10.1201/9781003748816-7

From the Artery the Blood rushes impetuously and per saltem by reason of the Dilatation and Constriction of the Heart, and is of a florid Colour. The Venal Blood flows with a more smooth and even Stream; it is of a grosser Consistence and of a darkish Colour [4].

In addition, he mentioned the valves of the veins, which are one of the vital components of Harvey's demonstration of circulation writing:

To which it may be added, that the Valves of the Vein... [5].

The first striking difference between Wiseman's book and the writings of his predecessors is the use of case histories. This facilitated the expression of the emotions associated with surgical therapy and the reactions of patient and surgeon to painful procedures. One dramatic example concerned a private soldier wounded during a battle near Truro in Cornwall. Wiseman wrote:

At the beating up of some of our Out-guards near Truro, the Enemy pursuing them, a Trooper, wounded between the Right Brow and Ear, espying me amongst the Crowd, importuned me earnestly to dress him, and would admit no Excuse. We stopt at an Apothecary's House on the Right Hand going out of the Town towards Perin. I call'd to the Apothecary's Servant to bring somewhat to dress him. Mean while I hastily lifted up the bloody Hair, and saw a Quantity of the Brain lie among it. I took it up with my Fingers, and shew'd it to him; the Sight whereof so calm'd his Passion, that I had Liberty to fly from the Enemy, who was enter'd the Town [6].

The courage and humanity of this report is most striking.

Pain of Surgery

Most of us are entertained by phenomena or behaviour that is contrary to what is expected. Wiseman exemplifies this with regard to a lady with a paronychia. (A paronychia is an inflammation located where the skin meets the side of a nail. It is excruciating.) Wiseman wrote:

A Gentlewoman came to my House one Night late, complaining exceedingly of a Pain in the pulp of one of her Fore-fingers. I looked upon it, and felt it hot, but saw nothing of Swelling whereby I could judge it so ill. She seem'd ready to swoon with the Pain. I proposed the making an Incision into it to the Bone: not imagining so fearful Creature would have permitted it; but she readily assented.... The next Day I waited upon her at her Lodging: she had slept well that Night, and in perfect ease [7].

There is relatively little in Wiseman's text about pain or fear of pain interfering with operations, though he did record cases where surgery was refused because of fear of pain. There is no criticism of this decision. There were two cases of children suffering from tuberculosis. One involved an eleven-year-old girl who had a cervical lymph node attached to the trachea. Before proceeding, this requires some explanations.

Tuberculosis is a disease caused by a bacterium. It mainly affects the lungs but may affect any organ in the body, including lymph nodes, especially in the neck.

Tuberculous inflammation of lymph nodes in the neck is essentially painless. Without treatment, it is very dangerous and ultimately lethal.

Bacteria are single-celled organisms without a nucleus. They can invade the body, multiply and do damage. They are treated with antibiotic medicines like penicillin. Tuberculosis is particular in this regard, as treatment usually is required for a long time (up to two years) and requires multiple antibiotics to be taken at the same time.

Lymphatic System. The lymphatic system consists of vessels separate from blood vessels. They drain excess fluid that leak into the tissues and carry it eventually back to the blood. It is a system of branching vessels and is interrupted by collections of cells called lymph nodes, which filter the lymph. In bacterial infections, the bacteria are caught up in the nodes and are attacked there by cells from the immune system. In consequence, during such infections the lymph nodes become swollen and tender. Tuberculous lymph nodes, while not tender, are swollen and stuck to surrounding tissues, requiring surgical removal.

Surgery was too painful for her, and had to be interrupted [8]. The other was a seven-year-old boy with advanced disseminated tuberculosis in multiple organs and tissues. One component of the disease was a dactylitis in the middle finger of his left hand. (Dactylitis is the inflammation of a digit, finger, or toe). Wiseman wanted to excise the finger but permission was not forthcoming [8].

Pain of Cautery

Wiseman had a few general comments on cautery not related to specific patients. One exception was his opposition to its use in the operations on hernias. His reason was that the procedures were hazardous and cruel. He seems to have had a preference for reporting cases where the result deviated from what was expected or advised. One example of this practice involved a patient with enlarged tonsils who refused actual cautery and was thus also treated with caustics, which shrank the tonsil, which was then ligatured and excised [9].

A thirty-five-year-old gentlewoman with a ranula had the lesion incised, and after drainage of fluid, it was cicatrized. (A ranula is a fluid-filled cyst that forms in the mouth, usually under the tongue, due to a damaged or blocked salivary gland.) However, subsequently it recurred, and this time actual cautery was used and was effective.

One case records the horrors of cautery and the courage of a gentleman of around fifty years of age. This unfortunate chap had cracked an apricot stone, which caused great pain in the teeth of his upper jaw. After a number of consultations, he was referred to Wiseman, who, with his colleagues, diagnosed an ulcerated cancer of the upper jaw. (The body's outer surface is covered by a tissue called skin. The tissue lining the gut and the airways is called the mucous membrane. An ulcer is a region where the surface tissue is missing, revealing diseased tissues beneath.) In Wiseman's case, the patient enquired how he was to be cured, and the doctors had not considered this as a possibility. Eventually, Sir Francis Prujean, who became president of the Royal College of Physicians answered that attempts at a cure were always unsuccessful and extremely painful, resulting in a shortening of the patient's life. The patient stated:

> *God's Will be done: I pray go and consider of the way; for I had rather die than live thus.*

A number of cauteries of various shapes were made together with instruments to protect the surrounding tissues. An assistant held the head and retracted the upper lip. Wiseman held the tongue down with a speculum, which is a metal instrument designed for that purpose. Having thus gained access, he proceeded to apply actual cautery to the upper jaw. He described the bone of the alveoli as 'rotten as dirt'. The patient became tired, and completion of the procedure was deferred until the next day. This involved cauterizing nearer to normal tissue, which was much more painful. Yet the patient sat cheerfully until the procedure was completed. At this point, he rose and washed out his mouth. The following days involved mouth washes and repeated cautery of any loose flesh. The patient survived around seven years, but a recurrence finally arose for which further treatment, including more actual cautery, was unsuccessful, and he languished and died.

Analgesics

With regard to painkillers, Wiseman revealed a change from earlier practice. For some patients, he prescribed oral opium-containing medicines for pain in the form of laudanum. This term had originally been coined by Paracelsus (1493 to 1541) for a tablet which included various obscure ingredients. One of the difficulties with taking oral opium is its bitter taste. However, Paracelsus found out that opium dissolved better in alcohol than in water, and he called the tincture so produced laudanum, from the Latin 'laudare', which means to praise. (A tincture is a solution in alcohol.) He also made a complex pill in addition to the tincture. There is a pharmacy in Prague which contains a laudanum powder inspired by the work of Paracelsus, and its constituents have been studied. They include extract of opium, saffron, crocus of the sun, pearls, horn of unicorn, red corals, clove oil, cinnamon oil, nutmeg oil, lemon oil, amber oil, amber, and musk [10].

A contemporary of Wiseman was the great physician Thomas Sydenham (1624 to 1689). Sydenham produced a tincture of laudanum by dissolving opium in sherry, which was much simpler than the complexities derived from the work of Paracelsus [11]. It is assumed that this was the preparation that Wiseman recommended for use for a patient with tongue cancer [12], for another sufferer with multiple ulcers and yet another with severe headache and multiple nodes and gummata (A gumma is a persistent local region of granulation tissue with a necrotic (see glossary) centre appearing in the late stages of syphilis) [13].

Finally, Wiseman was consistent in bowing to his patients' wishes when they refused proffered treatment, and he exercised himself in finding alternative means of management. There is no suggestion of an authoritarian approach to the treatment of pain.

It may also be mentioned that Wiseman did not record cases of bladder stone. He may well have left such cases to the excellent Thomas Hollier, whom he knew, and who famously operated on Samuel Pepys [1].

Phlebotomy

Wiseman's writings are about different diseases and injuries with accounts of how they were treated and what results were observed. It does not contain information on the techniques of treatment, including phlebotomy.

Conclusion

Wiseman moved in the highest social circles, yet when involved in trying to leave a battle, which his side was losing, he allowed himself to be detained to help a private soldier with a serious head injury. His reporting of cases in which advice was not followed or in which the result was unexpected illustrates his charming lack of omniscience. While Paré exercised himself to minimize the pain of cautery, he was nonetheless convinced of its value. Wiseman would seem to be the first surgeon who was beginning to doubt its value.

PIERRE DIONIS (1643 TO 1718)

Dionis was over twenty years younger than Wiseman and was born in the year King Louis XIV came to the throne of France. He was educated in the Confrérie de Saint-Côme. He entered that organization where the surgeons of the long robe had merged with the Barber-Surgeons in 1656. Thus, he was educated in a rather more distinguished organization than, for example, Ambroise Paré or Richard Wiseman. He became a famous teacher in the Royal Garden. This was an institution scientifically in advance of the University of Paris, and Harvey's teachings on the circulation of the blood were incorporated in the syllabus, in contrast with the rest of Paris [14]. He was highly regarded in Court circles, including the Dauphines and the Duchess of Burgundy among his clients [15].

He published a book in 1707 called 'A Course of Chirurgical Operations Demonstrated in the Royal Garden at Paris'. It was a text of major importance [16]. It is also the only guide we have to his character. The preface is a long essay on the superiority of surgery to almost any other activity, thereby emphasizing his importance in the scheme of things. He admitted that physicians were responsible for diseases that could not be cured by the knife. He accepted that they must supervise the activities of surgeons, but he clearly resented this and disliked physicians. He was also not particularly enamoured of his own profession, as will become apparent.

Fear of Surgery

On the one hand, Dionis was humane, concerned with minimizing the inevitable fear a prospective operation would induce. Dressings and equipment should not be delivered to a patient's home before the operation, since the sight of these instruments and dressings is terrifying. The surgeon should arrive with all the equipment he requires immediately before the operation is to be performed. He should then be quiet, calm, and affable to the patient. Also, the surgeon's work is not finished with the completion of the operation. He was responsible for the disorders consequent upon an operation, most especially bleeding and dressings [17]. Dionis' awareness of the pains of surgery is outlined in the beginning of his book:

> *There are Chirurgeons who are offended at the Cries of their Patients, who scold at and chide them, as though they ought to be insensible of the Tortures which they make them endure; these ways of acting are too cruel; a Chirurgeon must have Humanity,*

and exhort those under his hands to Patience: He must share their Pain; which, though he cannot help putting them to, he must, at least, leave them the Liberty of crying and complaining [17].

These are humane remarks, which are very much in keeping with the teachings of Celsus and Paré. Nonetheless, he has a self-righteous side, which is less attractive as expressed thus:

Some Authors have invented a Ring, in which they fix a small Incision Knife, which they make use of to open Abscesses in timorous Children, and such Persons as cannot be prevailed on to endure what they think proper to do to them: They put this Ring on one of their Fingers, and on pretence of feeling the Tumour, pierce it with the Incision Knife and so dextrously deceive their patients.

Dionis' response is:

But this Procedure seems to me to savour a little of the Mountebank; wherefore I can't advise you ever to make use of it. If this Operation is to be performed on a Child, it need only be held fast; and if any grown Person prove rank Coward enough not to suffer it, the Chirurgeon is to quit and abandon him to his Fate, without being at the trouble of searching after Stratagems to surprise him [18].

Dionis clearly believed he knew what pain was tolerable and he retained the right to judge those who disagreed with him.

Pain of Surgery

Nonetheless, despite his willingness to judge his fellows, he was, as stated above, humane and exercised himself to minimize the pain of a surgical operation. To this end, he insisted that knives and scissors should be kept sharp [19]. He also recommended that sutures should not be too long because the longer sutures would require more traction through the tissues, which would be painful [20]. Despite his contempt for what he viewed as cowardice, his respect for patients and his insight into behaviour are well illustrated in the next passage.

When a Chirurgeon has without hesitation acquainted the Patient that he must of necessity resolve to die, or undergo the Operation, there are none but will choose the Operation. We are not willing to die; and tho' we are certain of suffering great Pains, we always prefer them to Death. I have seen some press the proceeding to it so hard, that they would not allow Time for the Preparation of the Apparatus, and I have found others suffer it with Angelical Patience, which shews that there is nothing that Men will not endure to protract the last Hour [21].

His awareness of pain and how to cope with it is recounted in his advice on managing growing toenails.

This Operation, though but trivial, is yet very painful, insomuch that the Patients cannot endure it without crying out: But the Chirurgeon is not to be alarm'd by them, but taking

> *no notice of them he is to proceed on, and be very quick in the performance; for as soon as the piece of Nail is taken out, the Pain is over, and the Patient passes from a suffering Condition to Ease, which makes him forget his former Pain [22].*

He also had advice related to the difficulties of certain specific operations. Thus, he found that he could persuade patients to undergo thyroidectomy fairly easily, as it was not all that painful [23]. Unlike Wiseman, Dionis was familiar with lithotomy and included an adequate description of bladder stones and their treatments. There is a description of the methods of immobilization to maintain stability during painful surgery [24].

Some operations were painful, but from a modern point of view, they provided no benefit. Venepuncture was one such procedure. There was one other operation which provided no benefit and was much more painful. This was a clitorectomy, which had been a source of concern as early as in the works of Paul of Ægina [25], Albucasis [26], and Guy de Chauliac [27]. Henri de Mondeville included the topic in a list of subjects he planned to write about, but failed to achieve [28]. Dionis wrote as follows:

> *If the Clitoris does not extend outwards beyond the Bounds which Nature has prescrib'd it, there is no need of Operation, but sometimes it grows to a degree as to become as big and long as a Man's Yard; this happens frequently to the Ægyptian Women. The Europeans, who have this Part larger than other Women, are call'd Fricatrices, because they may abuse it and pollute themselves with other Women; which has made way for its Amputation, in order to deprive Women of a continual excitation to Lasciviousness: but there are very few who will submit to the Operation; for if a Woman be chaste she will not abuse it; and if debauch'd she will not voluntarily lose a Part which contributes to the Pleasure she enjoys in her Debauchery [29].*

The word 'yard' in this quotation is an archaic, obsolete term for 'penis'. Once again Dionis is adopting a tone of disapproval, which is by no means clearly justified.

Pain of Cautery

With regard to cautery, Dionis had this to say in principle.

> *I know no Chirurgeon which at present uses them, and tho' I have caused them to be engraven here, 'tis rather to excite Horror in you with regard to their Cruelty, than advise you to use them [30].*

In addition, in the section on Caesarean Section, he had this to say.

> *Good Chirurgeons have retrench'd the Fire from all Operations perform'd on the Flesh, and no longer make use of any more than a few burning Irons on those bones which are insensible, on which occasions also they are but rarely us'd. Our Art has abandon'd those harsh Methods by which Farriers torment with burning irons those poor Horses which they might otherwise cure: And if their way of making use of Irons and Fire strikes a horror into Spectators of this Practice on Animals, who is there could refrain complaining, who could see a Man's Belly burned, whose Cries would move the most stony Heart? [31].*

One example of the limited use of cautery on insensible bone is during the treatment of a lachrymal fistula. The fistula is first dilated and opened with a knife, after which cautery is applied to the bone [32]. Cautery was also used to dry up the ulcers of chronic atrophic rhinitis [33].

Analgesics

While much is written about minimizing pain, there is nothing in Dionis' text about specific analgesics.

Phlebotomy

Dionis presents and discusses the technique of phlebotomy in greater detail than any previous writer, which is reasonable since his book concerns the demonstration of operations.

With regard to the complications of phlebotomy, he wrote:

> *The greatest Misfortune is not that of making an Attempt without bleeding, but of opening an Artery, or pricking a Tendon. In which cases the Chirurgeon is never forgiven; for the World never examining the insurmountable Difficulties which occur in many Arms, nor the Risque which he runs in the undertaking of those forts of Bleedings, if he does not succed, when the Blame falls on him; for if he fails in Bleeding none will excuse him, or bear any Part of his Uneasiness; and to compleat his Misfortune, those who ought to defend him, are frequently tickled with a secret Rejoicing, and actuated by a jealous Temper are not displeas'd to see this Mortification fall on him [34].*

This is further evidence that he was prickly and self-involved.

He does not state plainly that pricking a tendon (or nerve) is very painful. Instead, he quotes Paré's experience with King Charles XI, mentioned in Chapter 6. He thus presents the symptoms of the complication as something recorded by someone else.

Conclusion

Dionis demonstrated a concern with maintaining surgical standards and minimizing the pain of surgery. He provides advice on multiple details of technique, the application of which reduces pain. In particular, he avoided the use of cautery simply because of the pain and fear it caused. All of this is ample evidence of the man's humanity. However, he exhibits a characteristic that seems to be specific for surgeons on the 'long robe' who have been educated in prestigious institutions of higher learning.

> *Three Dispositions of Mind are also requisite to the Patient who desires to be cured; namely, a great Share of Confidence, Patience, and Obedience; at the Instant that a Patient makes Choice of a Chirurgeon, he ought to believe that there are none more able than he; and to conform to that Persuasion, he must avoid harkening to those who propose to him imaginary Secrets, or particular Remedies, and abandon himself intirely to him; as chearfully rejoicing as though he saw his Health in the hands of him who is endeavouring to restore it to him [17].*

This is reminiscent of the attitudes of the medieval surgeons who received a university education, together with Peter Lowe, whose education had been of the same high formality (see Chapter 6). Humans are complex, so despite Dionis' evident humanity, kindness, and consideration, he preserved to himself the right to criticize those who do not live up to what he regarded as acceptable standards of behaviour.

DANIEL TURNER (1667 TO 1741)

Daniel Turner was born two years after the Great Plague of London and one year after the Great Fire. He was the son of John Turner, a member of The Tallow-Chandlers' Company of London. He trained at the Barber-Surgeons' Company of London from 1684 to 1691. In 1695, just three years after the end of his training and at the tender age of twenty-eight he published a book with the name 'Apologia Chyrurgica' [35], which is concerned with malpractice. The title page shown in Figure 7.1 shows how this book could have caused offense. Such bombastic utterances would not have been acceptable from someone of advanced years and would certainly have been resented

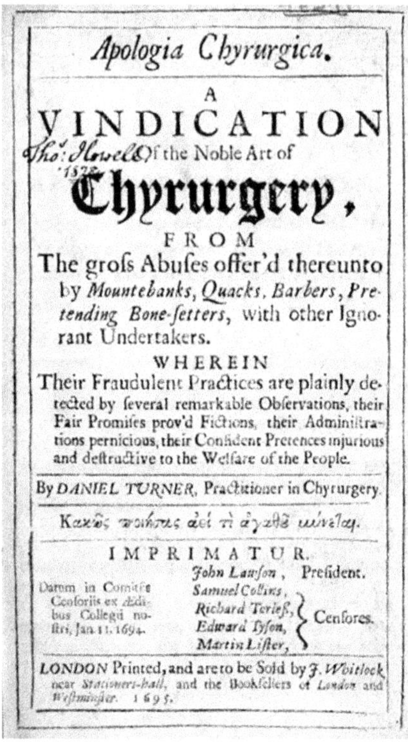
Apologia Chyrurgica.

A

VINDICATION

Of the Noble Art of

Chyrurgery,

FROM

The groſs Abuſes offer'd thereunto by *Mountebanks*, *Quacks*, *Barbers*, *Pretending Bone-ſetters*, with other Ignorant Undertakers.

WHEREIN

Their Fraudulent Practices are plainly detected by ſeveral remarkable Obſervations, their Fair Promiſes prov'd Fictions, their Adminiſtrations pernicious, their Confident Pretences injurious and deſtructive to the Welfare of the People.

By *DANIEL TURNER*, Practitioner in Chyrurgery.

[illegible]

IMPRIMATUR.

Datum in Comitiis Cenſoriis ex Ædibus Collegii noſtri, Jan. 11. 1694.

John Lawſon, Preſident.
Samuel Collins,
Richard Torleſs,
Edward Tyſon,
Martin Liſter, Cenſores.

LONDON Printed, and are to be Sold by *J. Whitlock* near *Stationers-hall*, and the Bookſellers of *London* and *Weſtminſter*. 1695.

FIGURE 7.1 Title page of Apologia Chyrurgica.

Three years after the end of his training, aged twenty-eight, he published this book on malpractice. The text on the cover portrays a lack of modesty and could easily have caused offense.

when uttered by a young man who could be reasonably assessed as a time-expired student.

In 1711, after thirteen years as a qualified surgeon, he paid £50 (around £8,200 in today's money) [36] to be released from the Barber-Surgeons' Company. He was a controversial figure, who had been described in a variety of ways. On the one hand, he was presented as a champion of professional standards in surgery and was critical of much that was current at the time [37]. His two-volume textbook 'Art of Surgery' was a systematic attempt to catalogue the diseases that were treated by surgery and the best way to achieve success [38].

Needless to say, such efforts could offend those whose practice he criticized. In his obituary at the Royal College of Physicians in London, it states:

> *Dr. Turner had some celebrity in his day; but was...too fond of displaying his talents upon paper; the result being that he published many volumes which are now forgotten. His cases...are not stated in the most delicate terms; nor was politeness amongst his excellencies [39].*

One can suspect that those words, to some extent, reflect the effect of tactlessness on physicians who would tend to look down on someone who was previously a surgeon. This patronizing attitude of physicians with regard to surgeons has persisted in Britain into modern times. Having practiced in the United Kingdom, Scandinavia, Austria, and Egypt, and taught in the United States, Mexico, and all over the Far East, it has become quite clear that retention of this attitude remains a particularly British unpleasantness. This view is confirmed by the quite different impression gained from a remark of that most distinguished surgeon, Percival Pott.

> *Dr. Daniel Turner compiled- a treatise of surgery, which was universally dispersed, and read all over the Kingdom, and was at that time generally looked upon as a true representation of the London practice [40].*

Another aspect of his character which could invite criticism was his aspiration to superior social standing. There is a picture of him in volume I of 'The Art of Surgery' which includes a motto which is identical to the motto of The Royal Society, (Nullius in Verba / *take nobody's word for it*) of which he was never a member or fellow (Figure 7.2).

Nonetheless, despite his weaknesses, his textbook on surgery is informative. In particular, like the work of Richard Wiseman, its value was increased by the numerous case histories. These are often detailed and long, even long-winded. He was clearly passionate about what he did, which, while resulting in every best effort for the patient, also included a wearisome tendency to emphasize his rightness and the errors of others. On the other hand, he was a critical thinker, openly questioning pneumatic theory, which was courageous since it challenged the accepted truth at the time. This theory was proposed by Galen, who taught that there were three kinds of spirit or breaths, called pneuma. One of these, called the animal spirit, was made in the brain and controlled its function. Turner's reflections on the animal spirit are mentioned below.

The following comment applied to a six-year-old boy who had been struck on the head by a stick thrown in a game which had missed its aim. He was struck on the 24th of February and died on the 23rd of May, during which time he was seen

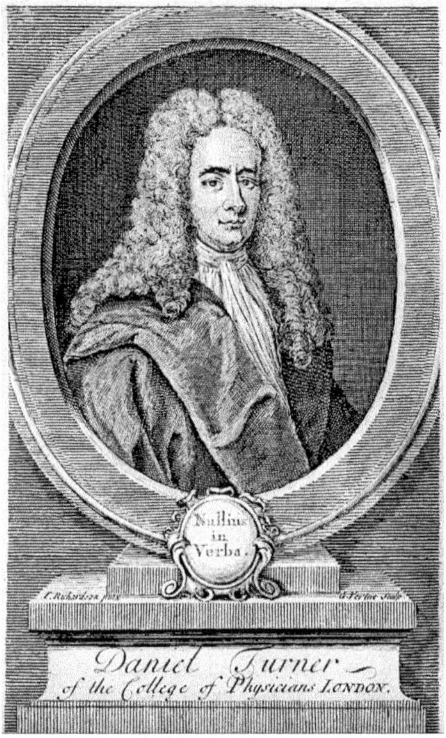
Nullius in Verba.
Daniel Turner
of the College of Physicians LONDON.

FIGURE 7.2 Image from the Art of Surgery (Vol 1).

This image in 'The Art of Surgery' includes the motto of the Royal Society (Nullius in Verba) to which Turner had no entitlement since he was never a member or a fellow.

repeatedly by Turner, who was deeply involved in his care. On his patient's death, Turner wrote:

> *Thus did the little Hero, of truly manly Courage, who struggled under, and got through so many Difficulties, and seemed now, in vulgar Estimation, to have been well and out of danger for a long time past, at last decease, after four-score and four Days.*

It turned out the child had an initially asymptomatic subdural abscess, which burst, causing the death. (The dura is the outermost of the three membranes that surround the brain inside the skull. In this patient, at autopsy, a localized collection of pus was found inside the dura between it and the brain. This is a subdural abscess.) Following this, Turner comments on his ignorance of the aetiology, and furthermore, could state:

> *Till the business of Sensation is better unravelled, than hitherto it hath been, or I fear will be; the Disorders of the nervous System may be conjectured, but not clearly demonstrated*
>
> *Whether there be any such Particles, as the animal Spirits, is not yet universally agreed on.*

These remarks illustrate both humanity and a willingness to question accepted doctrine. His varied reputation would seem to have resulted not only from undue arrogance but also from a passion that prevented him from being discrete in comments on practice of which he disapproved.

Pain of Surgery

Intense humanity shines through Turner's case histories, while he has little to say about the pain caused by the surgeon's knife. This is an important absence, as it shows that for an intense, emotional, and caring man, managing the pain of an operation was still not a high priority.

Pain of Cautery

There are many examples where Turner advocated the use of the actual cautery. In no instance does he consider the associated pain, indicating again that managing the pain of a procedure was not a high priority. He does, however, have some warning words related to the use of potential cautery. He advises the avoidance of more potent chemicals as follows:

> *I forbear mentioning some other Escharotics prepared from the several Arsenics or corrosive Sublimates, which I look upon as dangerous Medicaments, having frequently seen very unhappy Symptoms attending their Application, such as Spasms or Convulsions, from their malign Nature herby communicated to the nervous System, with horrid Pain, and Symptomatic Fever; also Cardialgia and incessant Vomiting, with cold Sweats, and Syncope or Fainting away [41].*

On a subsequent occasion, he relates the condition of a patient with cancer involving the mouth, lower jaws, and the neck. A colleague had prescribed a powerful caustic agent. Turner stops this on the grounds that it would have no beneficial effect, but would increase the pain from which the patient suffered [42]. His avoidance of powerful caustics applied not only to cancer but also to the treatment of wounds. He states:

> *For it is surely Hardship enough for the poor Patient to undergo the Pain and Smart from his Wound, with the unavoidable Symptoms attending, without the addition Torment occasion'd by many of these Escharotics, by which both Pain and Fluxion, as also Fever are excited, together with great Restlessness, and oftentimes convulsion [43].*

Finally, in contrast with the rather pompous opinion of Dionis about hiding the knife during the opening of abscesses, Turner approved of hiding cautery from women and children, writing:

> *That your Patient, especially if a Woman or Child, and more particularly a Woman with Child, be never suffer'd to see your Irons, or, if possible, to know any thing of them [44].*

Analgesics

There is occasional mention of opium and laudanum, but not in connection with the pain related to an operation.

Phlebotomy

Unsurprisingly, Turner warns of the possibility of pain arising from a badly performed phlebotomy, undertaken by someone whose qualifications he doubted.

> *To look, no farther than the Management even of a Lancet, what fatal Accidents have attended the opening of a Vein in the Arm; for which every ignorant Barber, now a Days, thinks himself well qualified? - Such I mean, as Punctures of the Tendon, from whence Pain, Convulsion, Apostemation, at some Times Gangrene or Mortification, at the best contracted Members, with stiff and almost useless Joints [43].*

He does not, however, describe the technique of phlebotomy, nor does he provide information about how to avoid this complication or how to treat the pain, should it arise.

Conclusion

Daniel Turner was able, passionate, and tactless with a desire for social advancement. He considered criticisms of surgeons by a lay public who lacked a surgeon's education to be necessarily unfair. His attitude that educated folk are superior is expressed at the beginning of his book, Apologia Chyrurgica where it is stated:

> *Tis the common Fate of Learned Men, that they are more than ordinarily expos'd to the importunity of such as are in want of their assistance [35].*

His attitude of social superiority led him to suggest the following behaviour from patients:

> *I could wish that every Patient would, make choice of such an honest and able Professor of this Art as they might reasonably confide in, and then wholly, under the Supreme Power, to submit themselves (without dictating their own erroneous Sentiments) to his management, I would -have them banish all those childish and fearful Apprehensions of his supposed Cruelty, and remain stedfast, in a firm belief, that he will act no otherwise by them than himself, if under such-like circumstances; or, that. what he does is purely design'd for their recovery and well being [35].*

This is reminiscent of medieval authoritarian attitudes mentioned earlier. It is also not unfair to note that his concern for suffering related to the illness prior to treatment and to the post-operative course. There is no question that everyone, patient, and surgeon accepted that the pain of surgery was unavoidable. Turner provides no evidence that there was a need to adapt the technique to reduce the suffering. But Turner was a man who had consistently and publicly criticized those with whom he did not agree, implying a very real sense of superiority. Another indication of his self-regard is the use of the first-person singular in his reports. He is one of only two surgeons mentioned in this book who used that format.

LORENZ HEISTER (1683 TO 1758)

Lorenz Heister was the son of a lumber merchant who later became an innkeeper and wine merchant [45]. Although not wealthy, his father was determined that he should have a university education [46]. He studied in a number of places, including Leyden, at the time of the celebrated clinical teacher Herman Boerhaave [47]. He obtained his degree at Herdewijk in 1708 [46, 48]. He was appointed to a variety of posts until settling in Helmstadt in 1719, where he was to stay for the rest of his life. In the same year, he published the first edition of his textbook 'Chirurgie'. This was not in Latin but in German, which he justified because the standard of education in Germany at the time was in a dreadful state [47]. Although the Thirty Years' War had ended in 1648, seventy-one years earlier, the social damage resulting from that war lingered on. It had been fought between mercenaries who lived off the land and who had inflicted appalling hardship on the civil population, which had still not really recovered [47, 49]. The book was translated into Latin eventually, and an English edition translated from the Latin was published in 1743. The systematic style and lucid prose made it a favourite [50]. Heister begins his text with an introduction which includes a mention of Celsus, for whom he clearly had the greatest respect.

> *...cures which are to be performed by the Hand, especially those which are attended with great danger and cruelty in the execution of them, require a singular hardiness of temper and resolution of mind, or as that "Cicero of the Physicians, Celsus, speaks", "An intrepid Mind void of all Tenderness and" Pity, and entirely deaf to the Shrieks and Outcries of the suffering Patients [51].*

PAIN OF SURGERY

Heister's concerns about pain and its avoidance are clearly expressed in the following passage about assessing whether indications for surgery exist in any given case.

> *Having finished his Examination, the next thing to be done is consider under what Class of Disorders it is to be ranked, and whether it be curable or not ? if it is deemed curable, whether it will be a Case of Time and Difficulty or not ? whether it is curable by Medicines alone ? or whether the Assistance of the Knife be necessary ? for the safest and most gentle Methods must always be preferred to harsh and dangerous ones, and are always to be tried first; but to Disorders of a violent nature, dangerous and even doubtful Remedies are to be tried. They are to be highly condemned therefore, who, after the Methods of " Mountebanks, condemn their Patients who labour under Hernia, without regard to Age or Habit of Body, to the Operation of the Knife, when far the greater part of them might be cured by a safer and easier Method, But if you shall find it impossible to save your Patient by gentle Methods, you should declare the Danger to the Patient, or rather to those about him, lest, if the Disorder should get the better of your Art, you should be suspected of being ignorant, or of having had an Intention to play the Rogue*

> *If the Surgeon shall find the Disorder to be curable, but to be of such a nature as to require the Knife, he should declare this in due time to the Patient, and should have his Approbation or Consent before he undertakes it; for a Surgeon is not only to take care to stop the Fury of the Disease, and lessen the present Pain, but also to provide against Accidents that may happen by delay; such as may chance to render the Case incurable. In very difficult Cases, the Surgeon not only provides for his Patient's Good, but his own, if he calls in other Physicians and Surgeons with whom he may consult before he proceeds to any Operation; for by this means he will save himself from all blame of having proceeded rashly or ignorantly, especially when he is concerned for Persons of Distinction, if things should go otherwise than he could wish [51].*

Finally, Heister adds the approach to the patient, preparing the operation to come.

> *When the Surgeon is entering upon the Operation, he ought to use his utmost Endeavours to encourage the Patient, by promising him in the softest Terms to treat him tenderly, and to finish with the utmost Expedition, and indeed he should use Expedition but not Hurry, and should be very careful to give no unnecessary Pain, but at the same time to leave no Mischief unremedied; if he observes these Rules, he will be sure to gain credit with the standers by [51].*

It is to be seen that he was most attentive to minimizing pain, and he also provides examples of how this principle may be achieved in practice. During limb amputation, applying a proximal tourniquet not only reduces haemorrhage by compressing the arteries but also reduces sensitivity to pain by compressing the nerves [52]. This is in keeping with the teachings of Paré mentioned in Chapter 6. Another detail which reduces pain is to use a knife to separate the periosteum of the bone so that it may be retracted proximally and avoid being cut by the saw, because it is pain sensitive [52].

He mentions the use of setons (see Chapter 6) and notes that opinion is divided as to their benefit. He himself thinks they can be useful, but qualifies that opinion after listing a large number of conditions, which he thinks may benefit from a seton:

> *But as Setons are usually attended with much Uneasiness and Trouble, their good Effects are but seldom experienced by Patients with those Disorders [53].*

If callous ulcers (chronic non-healing ulcers with a hard base and inelastic margins) were allowed to persist untreated for too long and milder treatments had failed, they would have to be excised, which was very painful. This is consistent with the above statement of risks arising if treatment is delayed [54].

Operating aneurysms was painful and dangerous and required care and circumspection, and should not be undertaken without the agreement and collaboration of other distinguished colleagues as noted above [55].

Two conditions affecting the nails of the fingers and toes are mentioned. Paronychia and ingrowing toenails absolutely require surgery, which is extremely painful. Paronychias may be of varying intensity, but they are dangerous because, if untreated, the inflammation may spread to the hand and even to the arm and, if further neglected, take the life of the patient. In view of these risks, the surgeon has a duty to convince the patient to undergo the necessarily painful operation. The pain is short lived and the benefits obvious [53]. The management of the ingrowing toenail makes no reference to the risks of the untreated condition and merely recommends surgery for relief of pain. Heister mentions that the surgery involving the use of strong nail scissors to cut free the offending nail is painful but only for a short time, followed by the benefit of pain relief [56].

Heister is concerned about the possibility of performing unnecessary surgery. One example he outlines is the castration of patients during hernia surgery. This he condemns as it causes avoidable pain and anxiety [57]. Another situation concerning the testis was a testicular swelling called a sarcocele. This required castration, and Heister noted that the procedure was less painful if the blood vessels to the testis were first ligated in the inguinal canal, close to the wall of the abdomen. The next step was to wait a few days until the testicle swelling decreased and the testicle consistency became more flaccid. This was less painful than ligating the blood vessels and removing the testis on the same day [58].

Heister mentions immobilization for more indications than any other surgeon. It was necessary for the following conditions. For paronychia, the whole arm had to be held still [53]. Two assistants held the head during cataract surgery [59]. An assistant held the head during trepanation [60]. In operations for tongue tumours, two assistants need to hold the tongue either with a cloth held between the fingers or with pliers [61]. During tracheotomy:

> *In the first Place, the Patient is to be inclined backward upon a Bed or in a Chair, and his Head held firm by an Assistant, who is to stand at his Back [62].*

A most unusual case by modern standards concerned a three-year-old child who had survived smallpox. However, advanced facial scarring had resulted in closure of the nostrils. An assistant held the hands and legs of the infant during the reopening of the passages of the nose.

There were also mentions of restraint by assistants in three operations in or near the abdomen. During surgery for bleeding piles, the legs must be held by two strong assistants [63]. During surgery for an inguinal hernia:

> *The Patient is first laid upon a Table, with his Head inclined backward, his Hips elevated, and all his Limbs and Head secured from moving, fastening them with Ligatures to the Table, or by holding with the Hands of Assistants [57].*

During a Caesarean Section:

> *… the Patient's Bladder should be emptied, least by distention it should be injured by the Knife, and the Patient then placed in the Middle of the Chamber upon the Bed, in such a Manner, that the Operator and his Assistants may each perform their proper Office: The Patient should then be encouraged with good and pious Words, and her Face covered from seeing the Instruments which might strike a Terror. And lastly, four strong Persons, at least, are to be placed to hold the Arms and Legs, that the Patient may not move under the Operation [64].*

That description underlines that births and thus Caesarean sections would be undertaken in the home with the poor woman lying on her bed.

The most detail about restraints is to be found in the description of how to undertake a lithotomy. It reads as follows:

> *It is generally necessary to provide three or four strong and courageous Assistants to secure the Patient firmly in a proper Posture for the Operation. Two of these Assistants are to secure the Patient's Legs on each Side, in such a manner as to hold his Foot fast in one Hand, and his Knee in the other, drawing it at the fame time to one Side. The third Assistant is to stand behind, and keep the Patient down on his Back close to the Table; and the fourth is to stand on the right Side of the Patient, or on the Table, in such manner as to hold up the Scrotum with one Hand, and to hold the Catheter, upon Occasion, with his other. A fifth Assistant may stand on the right Side of the Surgeon, that he may hold in Readiness, give and receive the several Instruments necessary for Lithotomy [65].*

It is hard not to be impressed by the precise thoroughness of Heister's instructions. Heister is also at pains to emphasize that lithotomy is difficult and dangerous and traditionally is usually performed by those who have special knowledge and expertise [65].

Heister also noted a variety of responses to patient fear. As mentioned above, in cases of paronychia, he made the extra effort to persuade the patient to permit surgery, in view of the serious consequences if the condition remained untreated. In addition, he opened tonsillar abscesses with a concealed lancet, in just the way Dionis had condemned [66].

For benign tumours that were large enough or hard enough to require surgery, if the patient refused, Heister recommended the use of caustic materials while at the same time expressing doubt as to the effectiveness of such treatments [67]. Again, he made the same recommendation when patients refused to have a hydrocele opened, though in this circumstance, he considered the caustic to be effective [68]. In the surgery of breast cancer, he met fearful women whose distress he said should be ignored, as stated by Celsus. On the other hand, he also mentioned women who bore the operation with courage and intrepidity [69].

Heister also refers to the operation of clitorectomy, but with a far more seemly and less moralistic tone than that employed by Dionis:

> *In some Women the Clitoris grows to so large a Size, as to equal and resemble the Penis of the male, upon which Account such Women have been called Hermaphrodites., notwithstanding the Clitoris is without any Perforation, and does not discharge either Semen or Urine. As the monstrous Size of this Part is a great Incumbrance to the conjugal Offices, the Surgeon's Assistance is therefore sometimes desired to remove the Impediment. This Disorder is said to have been frequent among the Arabians and Egyptians, insomuch that it was a common Practice with them to cut off the Part, which indecently appeared externally in the new-born Infant-, which, however, is an Operation seldom performed among the Europeans, because Women, who have this Part larger than usual, are desirous of concealing it, either through Lust, Modesty, or a Dread of the Knife [70].*

It is unclear why both Dionis and Heister associated clitoromegaly with the women of Egypt. There is no such mention in the writings of Paul of Ægina and the other earlier surgeons. Nor does modern literature lend support to the association [71, 72].

Pain of Cautery

While perhaps lacking the uncritical enthusiasm of some of his predecessors, Heister was by no means a complete opponent of the use of cautery. His attitude, as might be expected, is clearly expressed.

> *There are two Inconveniences which generally attend the use of Cautery, and sometimes force us to neglect it; for the first, not only the Patient is usually wonderfully terrified at the apprehension of it, but Mankind in general look upon it as a piece of Barbarity to advise the use of it; when, to say truth, it does not occasion such violent Pains as are usually apprehended from it, and what Pain there is in the Operation is instantly over [73].*

He defines the difference between actual and potential cauteries (see Chapter 2). He specifies that actual cautery may be used:

> *...to destroy dead Parts of carious bones, in Cancers, to remove schirri (hard lumps), Excrescences, Carbuncles and mortified Parts; but they are also used to make Issues and Setons, to stop Haemorrhages in Wounds and Amputations [74].*

With regard to using actual cautery to make issues (see Chapter 2), he admits that only a very few patients will permit this [75]. In the list of indications for cautery used as counterirritation, he includes:

> *...and lastly, to remove Amaurosis, Epilepsy, Sciatica, with Pins in the Teeth and other Parts [74].*

Heister mentions a number of caustic substances which may be used in potential cautery, but advises against the use of sublimates of arsenic and mercury as they are too likely to cause violent pains, convulsions, and even death [76].

While confirming his belief in the efficacy of cautery, he does not accept its indiscriminate use, and there are several examples of necessary precautions. In the first instance, it is necessary to protect adjacent tissues when cautery is applied to a diseased focus. This requires choosing a diathermy tip of the right shape and retracting adjacent normal tissues [74]. In actual cautery applied to a decayed tooth, every effort must be made to avoid the agony of applying the cautery to the surrounding gums [77]. It was also undesirable to use actual cautery for gum excrescences because that was too painful [78]. When cautery is used for a lachrymal fistula, the sound eye should be covered to avoid terrifying the patient [60]. Thus, if a patient refused the knife or actual cautery, potential cautery with appropriate caustics may be applied [67]. There have been a number of references to this practice, and it applies to the treatment of scrofula [79].

Heister introduced a welcome note of realism when discussing the relief of a toothache by applying actual cautery to a spot behind the ear. He proposed that the pain relief is due to fright, since he has observed a very intense toothache disappear at the mere sight of the cautery. Moreover, he affirmed that in his hands, the treatment often does not work and can thus not be the result of injuring some notional nerve that runs between the cautery location and the tooth. Damage to this non-existent nerve had been proposed by others as the mechanism by which pain relief was achieved. Heister was having none of it.

Finally, it may be noted that despite his belief in the efficacy of cautery, there were a variety of situations where he recommended caution. He believed that actual cautery is the most effective way of removing warts, which thereafter never return. However, he mentions that the treatment will occasion a most severe though brief pain [80].

Actual cautery was to be avoided in venomous wounds, as other methods were as effective, and there was no reason to torment the patient unnecessarily [81]. Penile warts could be successfully treated with potential cautery. If some remained, they could be removed with a knife or ligature. Actual cautery was considered too painful and severe in this condition [82].

Warts on the eyelids may be treated by ligature, knife, or caustics. Caustics must be applied extra carefully to ensure the eye is not damaged, with the risk of blindness. On no account must actual cautery be used, presumably for obvious reasons, although Heister does not specify what these might be [83]. Treatment is required when the eyelids are inverted so that the hairs on the eyelids irritate the underlying eye (Entropion). The recommended first stage of treatment was the mechanical extraction of each hair. This extraction should be done bit by bit to avoid unnecessary pain and inflammation. Cauterization of the roots has been attempted, but it is so painful that only a few patients will accept it, and so, potential cautery applied to the hair root holes is preferred [84].

An ancient term for any tumour arising in the mouth was 'Epulis' [85]. It is a term like schirrus, which is related to its appearance to the naked eye without having access to any examination under a microscope. Heister recommended that these lumps be best removed using a ligature or, if need be, the knife. He noted that some colleagues recommended actual cautery, but noted that using a cautery in the mouth is at best inconvenient. It is also extremely painful and should thus be avoided [78].

Finally, he forbade its use in the treatment of nasal polyps. He noted again that some colleagues use it, but he disagrees with the practice, since for the patient, the experience is torture, and there is a real risk of injuring normal parts of the nose [86].

Analgesics

Heister has no specific comments on the use of analgesics to reduce the pains of an operation.

Phlebotomy

As might be expected, Heister expressed himself with great clarity concerning the pains following injury to tendon or nerve during phlebotomy. He wrote:

> *What grievous and cruel Symptoms may arise from the pricking a nerve or Tendon, we have before intimated, in treating of Wounds... But you may reasonably judge, that a Nerve or Tendon has been injured in Bleeding, if the Patient, at the Time of Incision, feels a most acute Pain, so that he can scarce refrain from urging a severe Outcry; and, in a short time after, the excruciating Pains still continuing, the Limb swells, becomes inflamed, convulsed, stiff, and extended as in the Cramp; which Symptoms, if not timely relieved, threaten Convulsions of the whole Body, a Gangrene of the Part, and Death itself, in a short time [87].*

Conclusion

Heister was equipped with all the tact that Turner lacked. Of his relationship with patients, he wrote:

> *Lastly, that the Surgeon may not appear disagreeable or terrible to his Patients, especially if they are Persons of Distinction or Quality, he should diligently avoid the appearance of Roughness in his Behaviour, or Nastiness in his Dress: For good Breeding and Cleanliness have their proper Effect in all Parts of Life; but the Surgeon gains a particular Confidence with his Patient by his Address, which has no small share in the Success of his Endeavours [51].*

Moreover, having outlined the problem of coping with the pain of surgery as promulgated by Celsus, he goes on to state:

> *But at the same time, I would have him behave with such caution as to be guilty of no Act of Rashness or Cruelty, and very carefully avoid giving unnecessary Pain [51].*

He was exceptionally concerned about minimizing the pain of surgery as outlined in the above text. He gave the minimizing or avoidance of pain during surgery a higher priority than any previous surgeon.

HENRI FRANÇOIS LE DRAN (1685 TO 1770)

Little is known of Le Dran's personal background. On the title pages of two of his books published after 1745, a mention that he was a Fellow of the Royal Society is included [88, 89]. Apart from professional awareness of his qualities, his generous humanity is evidenced by his willingness to include management errors in his writings for the better enlightenment of those he taught.

Pain of Surgery

In the opening section of his book on operations, Le Dran was the first to suggest that operations should be expeditious to minimize the duration of inflicted pain. However, they should be undertaken effectively so that they adequately fulfil their aim. In addition, Le Dran wanted to know if a patient's condition was consistent with a good surgical result. He wrote as follows:

> *He ought in the next place to consider the age of his patient, his strength, and the state of his mind; and to judge from thence whether he is capable of supporting the fear, pain, and danger of the operation. Fear we know has a great effect upon the constitution, and we have seen instances of patients, who, immediately upon knowing there were no other means of cure than by an operation, have fallen into the most unhappy condition [90].*

His consideration for the comfort of the patient is demonstrated repeatedly. At the time, it was customary to drain abscesses through three incisions. By making two semicircular incisions meeting in the middle of the abscess, an adequate drainage opening is produced, involving two thirds the pain of the traditional three incisions

[91]. When draining a hydrocele, he found that making small perforations rather than incisions was more comfortable and also more effective [92].

When operating on a fistula in ano, using a blunt probe prevents the creation of new false passages and thus is more efficient at demonstrating the true course of the fistula [93].

When operating on piles, the technique should be altered according to the shape of the haemorrhoid. If it had a narrow base, then a ligature is the preferred treatment since there is no haemorrhage and when the ligature falls off, the patient is cured. On the other hand, if the base is broad, a knife is preferable, because the pain of a ligature applied over several hours is intolerable [94].

When trepanation is to be performed in the absence of a skin wound, an incision is needed. Le Dran preferred a 'T' shaped incision or an angular incision 'V' since they were simpler to manage and less painful than the traditional cruciate cut [95].

The method of immobilization is specified for surgery to the testis [96], fistula in ano [93], haemorrhoids [94], uvula excision [97], nasal polyp removal [98], and lithotomy [99]. With regard to lithotomy, he made two additional points. The surgeon needed to be prepared that patients who have accepted the need for lithotomy, on entering the premises where the operation is to be performed, could lose their courage and be plagued by all sorts of non-specific symptoms such as vomiting, diarrhoea, wind, and fever. It was also necessary to understand that the pain of surgery is unavoidable and may well last for an hour or more [99].

Pain of Cautery

This is limited in Le Dran's text as the use of cautery on soft tissues is considered too cruel [90]. There are a few mentions of the method in the book and, with two exceptions, they all recommend avoiding it. Le Dran considered that, while cautery of a lachrymal fistula could not be absolutely rejected, the method nonetheless terrified the patient, and the pain was so great that the technique had largely fallen into desuetude. On the other hand, potential cautery with a button of vitriol or alum may be used for haemostasis during amputation. However, Le Dran, where possible, preferred a ligature [100].

Analgesia

There is no mention of analgesic agents to reduce the pain of an operation.

Phlebotomy

Phlebotomy is mentioned, but there is no description of the technique and complications.

Conclusion

Le Dran provides specific examples of technical details of operations which will minimize the pain involved. He does not make any statement of principle regarding the personal behaviour of patients. His primary focus is teaching and the preservation of knowledge. He states:

> *Surgery owes its Rise to Observation; which has been since enriched by Reflection [101].*

> *The first thing that requires the surgeon's consideration, is to endeavour to gain a thorough knowledge of the disease entrusted to his care [90].*

> *There can be no young Surgeon but what is desirous of curing his Patient, either from Humanity, Honour, or Interest [102].*

While Le Dran was humane as shown above, his highest priority was attempting to improve and maintain the standard of his profession.

SAMUEL SHARP (1709 TO 1779)

Samuel Sharp was born in London on 17 July 1709. His father was Henry Sharp of Jamaica, and his mother was Hannah Puller, daughter of a previous Mayor of Hertford (103). Despite no university education, he was capable in Latin and French. Indeed, he had spent time in France, meeting Voltaire and gaining familiarity with French surgery. He was apprenticed to William Cheselden, starting when he was sixteen years old. He obtained his diploma from the Barber-Surgeons' Company in March 1732 and was elected surgeon to Guy's hospital in 1733 [103]. He was distinguished enough to be elected a fellow of the Royal Society and a foreign member of the Royal Academy of Surgery in Paris. In 1745, during his lifetime, the King granted a license for the formation of a Company of Surgeons, separate from the barbers. Sharp was on the Court of Assistants of the Company.

Sharp was well known for his talents as an eye surgeon, particularly his surgery for cataracts. He was consulted by Georg Friedrich Händel, who became blind in his later years. Sharp made no offer to operate because he could not see any evidence of a cataract [104]. Like Dionis and Le Dran, he was an opponent of the use of cautery. He wrote a textbook on the operations and instruments of surgery, in which he stated that:

> *In the Description of Diseases I have only mention'd their distinguishing Appearances, and have not once dared to guess at that particular Disorder in the Animal Oeconomy, which is the immediate Cause of them; indeed the Uncertainty there is in Conjectures of this intricate Nature, and the little Service that can accrue to Surgery from such speculative Enquiries, have entirely deterred me from all Pretence to this sort of Theory; and since the most ingenious Men hither to, have not by the help of Hypotheses, done any considerable Service to the Practice of Surgery, nay, for the most part have misled young Surgeons from the Study of the Symptoms and Cure of Diseases, to an idle turn of Reasoning, and a certain Stile in Conversation which has very much discredited the Art amongst Men of Sense; I hope I am right in my Silence on that Head [105].*

This is a statement reminiscent of Daniel Turner's comments on the nature of sensation. It shows a true scientific attitude with a scepsis directed to speculative notions not based on evidence. It is also a long single sentence containing 147 words; an unusual, surprisingly lucid excess.

Pain of Surgery

Sharp gave technical advice to reduce pain in three situations. He, like several predecessors, was concerned about the use of probes, advising that probing wounds could cause damage [106]. He advocated opening abscesses with a knife, as this was considerably less painful than using scissors. There were also situations where probing abscesses could tear them open, and this should be avoided [107]. Another important detail to prevent unnecessary pain concerned ligating haemorrhoids; advice that turned up unusually in a chapter on tonsils. Sharp, like Le Dran, was aware that when multiple ligatures were required in the treatment of haemorrhoids, the pain could be intolerable if all the ligatures were inserted at the same time. He advised that no more than two should be inserted together [108].

Like his predecessors, he repeated the need for immobilizing patients prior to surgery. He wrote details of how this should be achieved in operations such as castration [109] or lithotomy [110, 111].

Pain of Cautery

He advised that the use of caustics should be avoided since they served no useful purpose and were painful [112]. The opening of an abscess with a knife is less painful than the use of caustics. Nonetheless, another reason for their use is when a patient refuses the knife. However, he admits that while caustics are more painful than the knife, they are to be preferred when the skin is thin and inflamed. In this situation, using the knife alone runs the risk that small sinuses would form and burrow under the lips of the incision. Use of the caustic prevents this complication [107].

There was one other application of potential cautery which he criticized. Applying caustics to ulcers in bones where the underlying bone is carious had no useful function. The only acceptable technique was the removal of the carious bone. In addition, he abhorred the use of actual cautery to accelerate the exfoliation of diseased bone at the base of ulcers [113]. He concluded the introduction to his book with the remark that actual cautery applied to naked bone every day is never useful and always cruel and painful. In consequence, for the most part, it had fallen into disuse.

There is one other comment on the ills of cautery. He referred to surgery for inguinal hernias, where it has been the practice following reduction of the intestine back into the abdomen, to destroy the skin over the rings of the abdominal muscles with actual cautery. This had the disadvantage that with recurrent hernia, the risk of strangulation is increased. Moreover, the success of the operation did not justify the pain [114].

Analgesics

There is no mention of the use of analgesics to reduce the pain of an operation.

Phlebotomy

There is no description of the technique of phlebotomy and no mention of related complications.

Conclusion

The title of Sharp's book is:

> *A Treatise on the Operations of Surgery, With a Description and Representation of the Instruments Used in Performing Them. To Which is Prefixed an Introduction on the Nature and Treatment of Wounds, Abscesses and Ulcers [115].*

It is about the practicalities of surgical technique. It avoids detail analysis of clinical pictures and indications. His intense dislike of cautery is a measure of his humanity, but the book contains no remarks about behaviour, either of the surgeon or of the patient.

SUMMARIZATION

During this period, anatomy studies were on a much firmer footing following the revolutionary work of Vesalius, ensuring more accurate planning and dissection during operations. While Harvey introduced the circulation of the blood during this period, this did not yet have the impact it would have in the future. Bloodletting remained popular, although the mentions of the pain or discomfort involved were very uneven. While variously expressed, there does seem to have been an increasing effort to minimize pain and an increasing willingness to accept patients' refusal to accept painful procedures which were not absolutely necessary. Nonetheless, the management of the pains of surgery remained similar to that defined by Celsus during the Roman Empire (see Chapter 3). This was mentioned repeatedly and paraphrased throughout the period.

REFERENCES

1. Wiseman R. *Oxford Dictionary of National Biography*. Oxford: Oxford University Press; 2008.
2. Ellis H. Richard Wiseman: The Best Known English Surgeon of the 17th Century. *British Journal of Hospital Medicine*. 2020; 81(11): 1–2.
3. Smith AD. Richard Wiseman: His Contributions to English Surgery. *Bulletin of the New York Academy of Medicine Journal*. 1970; 46(3): 167–82.
4. Wiseman R. *Treatise V. Chapter II Of Wounds of the Veins and the Arteries. Eight Chirurgical Treatises*. London: Walthoe, J et al; 1734, pp. 63–70.
5. Wiseman R. *Treatise V of Wounds. Chapter XIV Of a Varix. Eight Chirurgical Treatises. I*. London: Walthoe, J et al; 1734, pp. 106–9.
6. Wiseman R. *Treatise V of Wounds. Chapter IX Of Wounds of the Head. Eight Chirurgical Treatises. II*. London: Walthoe, J et al; 1734, pp. 105–49.
7. Wiseman R. *Treatise I of Tumours. XI Paronychia. Eight Chirurgical Treatises. I*. London: Walthoe, J et al; 1734, pp. 90–7.
8. Wiseman R. *Treatise IV Of the KING'S EVIL. Eight Chirurgical Treatises. I*. London: Walthoe, J et al; 1734, pp. 392–511.

9. Wiseman R. *Treatise IV Chapter VII Of the Tonsils. Eight Chirurgical Treatises. II.* London: Walthoe, J et al; 1734, pp. 31–6.
10. Nesměrák K, Šticha M, Beliansky M, Červený V, Kozlik P, Kudláček K, et al. Laudanum Opiatum Caesareum: Authentication of the Composition of a Historical Pharmaceutical Preparation from the Eighteenth Century Using a Multianalytical Approach. *Monatshefte für Chemie*. 2021; 152: 1089–96.
11. Sydenham T. *Dictionary of Medical Biography*. Westport, CT: Greenwood Press; 2007, pp. 1209–12.
12. Wiseman R. *Of a Cancer. Eight Chirurgical Treatises. I.* London: Walthoe, J et al; 1734, p. 193.
13. Wiseman R. *Treatise VIII Of Lues Venerea. Of the Cure of Symptoms. Eight Chirurgical Treatises. II.* London: Walthoe, J et al; 1734, pp. 327–89.
14. Tubbs RS, Groat C, Loukas M, Shoja MM, Ardalan MR, Cohen-Gadol AA. Pierre Dionis (1643-1718) Surgeon and Anatomist. *Singapore Medical Journal*. 2009; 50(4): 447–9.
15. Dionis P. (Ed.). *Dictionary of Medical Biography*. London: Greenwood Press; 2007, pp. 419–20.
16. Simpson D. Pierre Dionis and the Franco-British Dialogue in Surgery. *ANZ Journal of Surgery*. 2003; 73: 336–40.
17. Dionis P. *Of Operations in General A Course of Cirurgical Operations*. London: Jacob Tonson; 1710, pp. 1–11.
18. Dionis P. *Of the opening of an Abscess A Course of Cirurgical Operations*. London: Jacob Tonson; 1710, pp. 454–61.
19. Dionis P. *Chirurgical Instruments. A Course of Cirurgical Operations*. London: Jacob Tonson; 1710, pp. 11–6.
20. Dionis P. Of Gastrorhaphy. In *A Course of Cirurgical Operations*. London: Jacob Tonson; 1710, pp. 49–58.
21. Dionis P. Of the Bubonocele. In *A Course of Cirurgical Operations*. London: Jacob Tonson; 1710, pp. 188–96.
22. Dionis P. Of the Nail growing into the Flesh. In *A Course of Cirurgical Operations*. London: Jacob Tonson; 1710, pp. 430–40.
23. Dionis P. Of the Goetre. In *A Course of Cirurgical Operations*. London: Jacob Tonson; 1710, p. 353.
24. Dionis P. Of the Operations Practised on the Bladder, Yard and Matrix. In *A Course of Cirurgical Operations*. London: Jacob Tonson; 1710, pp. 98–123.
25. Adams F. On Extirpation of the Nympha and Cauda Pudendi. In *The Seven Books of Paulus Æginata. II.* London: The Sydenham Society; 1846, p. 381.
26. Albucasis. On Cutting the Clitoris and Fleshy Growths in the Female Genitalia. In *Albucasis on Surgery and Instruments - A Definitive Edition of the Arabic Text with English Translation and Commentary*. Berkeley, CA: University of California Press; 1973, p. 456.
27. de Chauliac G. Diseases of the Matrix. In *The Major Surgery of Guy de Chauliac: An English Translation*. Bloomington, IN: XLibris; 2007, p. 562.
28. De Mondeville H. The Descriptive Rubrics for the 43 Chapters he planned for his Doctrine III are in Vol. II, Part II and fill 6 pages. In *The Surgery of Henri de Mondeville. II.* Bloomington, IN: XLibris; 2003, pp. 915–23.
29. Findlen P. *A History of the Male and Female Genitalia 2000*. Available from: https://web.stanford.edu/class/history13/earlysciencelab/body/femalebodypages/genitalia.html#:~:text=%22The%20uterus%20is%20called%20also,a%20cold%20and%20dry%20organ

30. Dionis P. Of Cauteries. In *A Course of Cirurgical Operations*. London: Jacob Tonson; 1710, pp. 466–70.
31. Dionis P. Of the Cæsarean Section. In *A Course of Cirurgical Operations*. London: Jacob Tonson; 1710, pp. 86–97.
32. Dionis P. For the Corners of the Eyes. In *A Course of Cirurgical Operations*. London: Jacob Tonson; 1710, pp. 307–12.
33. Dionis P. *Of the Polypus*. In *A Course of Cirurgical Operations*. London: Jacob Tonson; 1710, pp. 313–22.
34. Dionis P. Of the Bleeding, and All that Belongs to It. In *A Course of Cirurgical Operations*. London: Jacob Tonson; 1710, pp. 357–82.
35. Turner D. *Apologia Chyrurgica*. London: J. Whitlock; 1695.
36. Anon. *Bank of England Inflation Calculator 2025*. Available from: https://www.bankofengland.co.uk/monetary-policy/inflation/inflation-calculator
37. Jenner M. Turner, Daniel. In: Bynum WBH, editor. *Dictionary of Medical Biography T-Z*. London: Greenwood Press; 2007, pp. 1247–8.
38. Wilson PK. Daniel Turner and the Art of Surgery in Early Eighteenth-Century London. *The Journal of the Royal Society of Medicine*. 1994; 87(December): 781–5.
39. Munk W. *Daniel Turner* London: Royal College of Physicians; 2009. Available from: http://munksroll.rcplondon.ac.uk/Biography/Details/4504
40. Pott P. *Observations on that Disorder of the Corner of the Eye Commonly called Fistula Lachrymalis*. 2nd ed. London: L. Hawes and Co.; 1763.
41. Turner D. Of the Diverse Kinds of Caustics, and the Manner of Applying Them. In *The Art of Surgery. I*. London: Rivington, C; 1736, pp. 22–4.
42. Turner D. Of the Cancer, its Cause, Signs and Cure. In *The Art of Surgery. I*. London: Rivington, C; 1736, pp. 80–99.
43. Turner D. Of Wounds in General. In *The Art of Surgery. I*. London: Rivington, C; 1736, pp. 326–99.
44. Turner D. Wounds of the Veins and Arteries. In *The Art of Surgery. I*. London: Rivington, C; 1736, pp. 525–40.
45. van der Pas PW. *Heister, Lorenz 2018*. Available from: https://www.encyclopedia.com/people/medicine/medicine-biographies/lorenz-heister
46. Zimmerman L, Veith I, Lorenz H. *Great Ideas in the History of Surgery*. New York: Dover Publications; 1967, pp. 313–23.
47. Stewart J. Lorenz Heister: Surgeon. *The Canadian Medical Association Journal*. 1929; 20(4): 418–9.
48. Heister L. *Dictionary of Medical Biography*. London: Greenwood Press; 2007, pp. 625–6.
49. Anon. *Mercenaries in the Thirty Years' War - Horrid Men or Great Soldiers?* 2021. Available from: http://www.historyisnowmagazine.com/blog/2021/10/18/mercenaries-in-the-thirty-years-war-horrid-men-or-great-soldiers#:~:text=The%20mercenary%20is%20often%20forgotten,commanders%20such%20as%20Gustavus%20Adolphus
50. Heister L. *A General System of Surgery in Three Parts*. London: W Innys; 1743.
51. Heister L. Introduction. In *A General System of Surgery in Three Parts. 1*. London: W Innys; 1743, pp. 1–25.
52. Heister L. Amputation of the Hand, Humerus and Cubitus. In *A General System of Surgery in Three Parts. I*. London: W Innys; 1743, pp. 334–40.
53. Heister L. Of the Paronychia. In *A General System of Surgery in Three Parts. 2*. London: W Innys; 1743, pp. 267–74.
54. Heister L. Of Ulcers. In *Book IV Chapter Callous Ulcers. A General System of Surgery in Three Parts. 1*. London: W Innys; 1743, pp. 251–2.

55. Heister L. Of Aneurisms. In *A General System of Surgery in Three Parts. 1*. London: W Innys; 1743, pp. 290–303.
56. Heister L. The Method of cutting out the Nail of the Great-toe, when it turns into the Flesh. In *A General System of Surgery in Three Parts. 2*. London: W Innys; 1743, pp. 287–8.
57. Heister L. Of the Enterocele. In *A General System of Surgery in Three Parts. 2*. London: W Innys; 1743, pp. 56–61.
58. Heister L. Of spurious Ruptures, and first of the Sarcocele, and Castration. In *A General System of Surgery in Three Parts. 2*. London: W Innys; 1743, pp. 63–5.
59. Heister L. Of Cataracts, or Suffusions. In *A General System of Surgery in Three Parts. I*. London: W Innys; 1743, pp. 402–16.
60. Heister L. Of Operations in the Head. In *A General System of Surgery in Three Parts. 1*. London: W Innys; 1743, pp. 351–476.
61. Heister L. Of a Scirrhus and Cancer under the Tongue. In *A General System of Surgery in Three Parts. I*. London: W Innys; 1743, pp. 467–8.
62. Heister L. Of Bronchotomy, or Laryngotomy, more properly termed Tracheotomy. In *A General System of Surgery in Three Parts. 2*. London: W Innys; 1743, pp. 4–7.
63. Heister L. Of the Bleeding Piles. In *A General System of Surgery in Three Parts. 2*. London: W Innys; 1743, pp. 248–9.
64. Heister L. Of the Caesarean Section or Birth. In *A General System of Surgery in Three Parts. 2*. London: W Innys; 1743, pp. 26–36.
65. Heister L. Of Lithotomy by the Apparatus minor, and of nephrotomy. In *A General System of Surgery in Three Parts. 2*. London: W Innys; 1743, pp. 101–9.
66. Heister L. Of opening Abscesses in the Tonsils. In *A General System of Surgery in Three Parts. I*. London: W Innys; 1743, p. 472.
67. Heister L. Of Encysted Tumours, whether, Schirrhus, Steatorma, Atheroma, or Meliceris. In *A General System of Surgery in Three Parts. 1*. London: W Innys; 1743, pp. 323–7.
68. Heister L. Of the Hydrocele. In *A General System of Surgery in Three Parts. 2*. London: W Innys; 1743, pp. 65–70.
69. Heister L. Of the Cancer in the Breasts. In *A General System of Surgery in Three Parts. 2*. London: W Innys; 1743, pp. 13–6.
70. Heister L. Of an Enlarged Clitoris. In *A General System of Surgery in Three Parts. 2*. London: W Innys; 1743, p. 197.
71. Soto AL, Gonzalez MB, Reyes MU, Jimenez LCM, Sanchez AB, Morcillo JG, et al. Imaging in fetal genital anomalies. *European Journal of Obstetrics and Gynecology and Reproductive Biology*. 2023; 283: 13–24.
72. Williams CE, Nakhal RS, Achermann JC, Creighton SM. Persistent Unexplained Congenital Clitoromegaly in Females Born Extremely Prematurely. *Journal of Pediatric Urology*. 2013; 9(6).
73. Heister L. Of the Accidents or Symptoms of Wounds. In *A General System of Surgery in Three Parts. 1*. London: W Innys; 1743, pp. 45–51.
74. Heister L. Of actual Cauteries. In *A General System of Surgery in Three Parts. 1*. London: W Innys; 1743, pp. 318–9.
75. Heister L. Of Issues. In *A General System of Surgery in Three Parts. 1*. London: W Innys; 1743, pp. 314–6.
76. Heister L. *Of Caustic and Corroding Medicines*. In *A General System of Surgery in Three Parts. 1*. London: W Innys; 1743, pp. 320–1.
77. Heister L. Of Hollow and Decayed Teeth. In *A General System of Surgery in Three Parts. I*. London: W Innys; 1743, p. 458.

78. Heister L. Of Epulides or Excrescences of the Gums. In *A General System of Surgery in Three Parts. I.* London: W Innys; 1743, p. 463.
79. Heister L. Of strumous or schrophylous Tumors and Bronchocele. In *A General System of Surgery in Three Parts. 2.* London: W Innys; 1743, pp. 7–9.
80. Heister L. Of Warts. In *A General System of Surgery in Three Parts. 1.* London: W Innys; 1743, pp. 321–2.
81. Heister L. Of Venomous Wounds and those that are made by the Bites of Animals. In *A General System of Surgery in Three Parts. 1.* London: W Innys; 1743, pp. 97–102.
82. Heister L. Of Warts, and other Excrescences of the Penis. In *A General System of Surgery in Three Parts. 2.* London: W Innys; 1743, pp. 82–3.
83. Heister L. Of Warts on the Eye-lids. In *A General System of Surgery in Three Parts. I.* London: W Innys; 1743, p. 367.
84. Heister L. Of Trichiasis, or Inverstion of the Eye-Lids; in whith the Hairs irritate the Eyes. In *A General System of Surgery in Three Parts. I.* London: W Innys; 1743, pp. 369–70.
85. Epulis. *Black's Medical Dictionary.* 39th ed. Lanham, MD: Madison Books; 1999.
86. Heister L. Of a Polypus in the Nose. In *A General System of Surgery in Three Parts. I.* London: W Innys; 1743, pp. 436–44.
87. Heister L. Puncture of a Nerve or Tendon. In *A General System of Surgery in Three Parts. 1.* London: W Innys; 1743, pp. 286–7.
88. Le Dran H-F. *Observations in Surgery; Containing One Hundred and Fifteen Different Cases; With Particular Remarks on Each, for the Improvement of Young Students.* London: J Hodges at the Looking Glass; 1740.
89. Le Dran H-F. *The Operations in Surgery.* London: C. Hitch; 1749.
90. Le Dran H-F. *Introduction. The Operations in Surgery.* London: J Hodges at the Looking Glass; 1749, pp. 1–9.
91. Le Dran H-F. Of an Inflammation. In *The Operations in Surgery.* London: J Hodges at the Looking Glass; 1749, pp. 9–27.
92. Le Dran H-F. Of Dropsies. In *The Operations in Surgery.* London: J Hodges at the Looking Glass; 1749, pp. 112–41.
93. Le Dran H-F. Of the Fistula in Ano. In *The Operations in Surgery.* London: J Hodges at the Looking Glass; 1749, pp. 158–72.
94. Le Dran H-F. Of the Haemorrhoids.In *The Operations in Surgery.* London: J Hodges at the Looking Glass; 1749, pp. 173–84.
95. Le Dran H-F. Of Wounds of the head. In *The Operations in Surgery.* London: J Hodges at the Looking Glass; 1749, pp. 368–98.
96. Le Dran H-F. Of the Diseases of the Testicles. In *The Operations in Surgery.* London: J Hodges at the Looking Glass; 1749, pp. 142–9.
97. Le Dran H-F. Of the Quincy. In *The Operations in Surgery.* London: J Hodges at the Looking Glass; 1749, pp. 323–39.
98. Le Dran H-F. Of the Polypus. In *The Operations in Surgery.* London: J Hodges at the Looking Glass; 1749, pp. 346–56.
99. Le Dran H-F. Of the Stone. In *The Operations in Surgery.* London: J Hodges at the Looking Glass; 1749, pp. 185–270.
100. Le Dran H-F. Of Amputations. In *The Operations in Surgery.* London: J Hodges at the Looking Glass; 1749, pp. 422–44.
101. Le Dran H-F. *To All Young Students in Surgery. Observations in Surgery; Containing One Hundred and Fifteen Different Cases; With Particular Remarks on Each, for the Improvement of Young Students.* London: J Hodges at the Looking Glass; 1740, pp. i–vi.

102. Le Dran H-F. Preface. *Consultations of most of the Disorders That Require the Assistance of Surgery*. London: Robert Horsfield; 1766, pp. vii–xvi.
103. Kirkup J. Samuel Sharp and the Operations of Surgery, 1739. *Journal of Medical Biography* 1996; 4: 1–7.
104. Jackson DM. Bach, Handel and the Chevalier Taylor. *Medical History*. 1968; 12(4): 385–93.
105. Sharp S. Preface. In *A Treatise on the Operations of Surgery, With a Description and Representation of the Instruments Used in Performing Them To Which is Prefixed an Introduction on the Nature and Treatment of Wounds, Abscesses and Ulcers*. London: J. Brotherton, W. Innys, R. Manby, J.&P. Knapton, C.Rivington, T. Longman, S. Birt, C. Hitch, S. Austen J. Hodges and G. Hawkins; 1739.
106. Sharp S. Of the Empyema. In *A Treatise on the Operations of Surgery, With a Description and Representation of the Instruments Used in Performing Them To Which is Prefixed an Introduction on the Nature and Treatment of Wounds, Abscesses and Ulcers*. London: J. Brotherton, W. Innys, R. Manby, J.&P. Knapton, C.Rivington, T. Longman, S. Birt, C. Hitch, S. Austen J. Hodges and G. Hawkins; 1739, pp. 115–25.
107. Sharp S. Of Inflammation and Abscesses. In *A Treatise on the Operations of Surgery, With a Description and Representation of the Instruments Used in Performing Them To Which is Prefixed an Introduction on the Nature and Treatment of Wounds, Abscesses and Ulcers*. London: J. Brotherton, W. Innys, R. Manby, J.&P. Knapton, C.Rivington, T. Longman, S. Birt, C. Hitch, S. Austen J. Hodges and G. Hawkins; 1739, pp. vii–xxviii.
108. Sharp S. Of the Extirpation of the Tonsils. In *A Treatise on the Operations of Surgery, With a Description and Representation of the Instruments Used in Performing Them To Which is Prefixed an Introduction on the Nature and Treatment of Wounds, Abscesses and Ulcers*. London: J. Brotherton, W. Innys, R. Manby, J.&P. Knapton, C.Rivington, T. Longman, S. Birt, C. Hitch, S. Austen J. Hodges and G. Hawkins; 1739, pp. 188–91.
109. Sharp S. Of Castration. In *A Treatise on the Operations of Surgery, With a Description and Representation of the Instruments Used in Performing Them To Which is Prefixed an Introduction on the Nature and Treatment of Wounds, Abscesses and Ulcers*. London: J. Brotherton, W. Innys, R. Manby, J.&P. Knapton, C.Rivington, T. Longman, S. Birt, C. Hitch, S. Austen J. Hodges and G. Hawkins; 1739, pp. 47–54.
110. Sharp S. Of the Greater Apparatus or the Old Way. In *A Treatise on the Operations of Surgery, With a Description and Representation of the Instruments Used in Performing Them To Which is Prefixed an Introduction on the Nature and Treatment of Wounds, Abscesses and Ulcers*. London: J. Brotherton, W. Innys, R. Manby, J.&P. Knapton, C.Rivington, T. Longman, S. Birt, C. Hitch, S. Austen J. Hodges and G. Hawkins; 1739, pp. 87–9.
111. Sharp S. Of the High Operation. In *A Treatise on the Operations of Surgery, With a Description and Representation of the Instruments Used in Performing Them To Which is Prefixed an Introduction on the Nature and Treatment of Wounds, Abscesses and Ulcers*. London: J. Brotherton, W. Innys, R. Manby, J.&P. Knapton, C.Rivington, T. Longman, S. Birt, C. Hitch, S. Austen J. Hodges and G. Hawkins; 1739, pp. 89–93.
112. Sharp S. Of Wounds. In *A Treatise on the Operations of Surgery, With a Description and Representation of the Instruments Used in Performing Them To Which is Prefixed an Introduction on the Nature and Treatment of Wounds, Abscesses and Ulcers*. London: J. Brotherton, W. Innys, R. Manby, J.&P. Knapton, C.Rivington, T. Longman, S. Birt, C. Hitch, S. Austen J. Hodges and G. Hawkins; 1739, pp. i–vii.

113. Sharp S. Of Ulcers. In *A Treatise on the Operations of Surgery, With a Description and Representation of the Instruments Used in Performing Them To Which is Prefixed an Introduction on the Nature and Treatment of Wounds, Abscesses and Ulcers.* London: J. Brotherton, W. Innys, R. Manby, J.&P. Knapton, C.Rivington, T. Longman, S. Birt, C. Hitch, S. Austen J. Hodges and G. Hawkins; 1739, pp. xxviii–xlix.
114. Sharp S. Of the Bubonocele. In *A Treatise on the Operations of Surgery, With a Description and Representation of the Instruments Used in Performing Them To Which is Prefixed an Introduction on the Nature and Treatment of Wounds, Abscesses and Ulcers.* London: J. Brotherton, W. Innys, R. Manby, J.&P. Knapton, C.Rivington, T. Longman, S. Birt, C. Hitch, S. Austen J. Hodges and G. Hawkins; 1739, pp. 11–25.
115. Sharp S. *A Treatise on the Operations of Surgery, With a Description and Representation of the Instruments Used in Performing Them. To Which is Prefixed an Introduction on the Nature and Treatment of Wounds, Abscesses and Ulcers.* London: J. Brotherton, W. Innys, R. Manby, J.&P. Knapton, C.Rivington, T. Longman, S. Birt, C. Hitch, S. Austen J. Hodges and G. Hawkins; 1739.

8 Surgical Pain – Transition to the Nineteenth Century: James Latta (1754–1804)

Five surgeons are to be considered in this chapter and its successors. Four of them were from Scotland, which at the beginning of the eighteenth century, was a small and impoverished country [1, 2]. Its southern neighbour, England, with which it had been on a collision course for centuries, was wealthy, advanced, and prosperous. Yet it was in impecunious Scotland that important advances in surgery and its education were to develop. There were a number of reasons. Firstly, while most unpopular at the time, the Act of Union of 1707 joined the two countries under one crown. This gave the Scots access to English institutions and trading advantages with a concomitant improvement in the standard of living. This was confirmed at the time by a Scottish aristocrat William Mackintosh, Laird of Borlum (1658–1743), who in 1715 had led a rebellion to replace the King of England with a descendant of the Scottish family that had ruled both countries since 1603. While he was clearly not in favour of the English nor of the Union, in 1729 he wrote:

> *In every mouth we hear the country is mightily improved since the Union.' And if you ask wherein, you are told 'If I don't see how much more handsomely the gentry live now than before' the Union in dress, table and house furniture?... This epidemick, this increase of spending-but to be modish and well-bred, I ought to have said this new improvement-has in these 20 years strangely over-run the nation in the very remotest corners [1].*

So, the Union may not have been universally popular, but it was improving the standard of living in Scotland as viewed by Scots. At the same time, an intellectual revolution was developing in Scotland that came to be known as the Scottish Enlightenment, which was based mainly in Edinburgh [3]. One of the benefits that accrued from this was a significant advance in medical and surgical education. The details of the advances may be found elsewhere [2, 4]. These improved standards attracted students. Two other factors also contributed. Firstly, Herman Boerhaave, in Leyden, the great founder of clinical teaching, died in 1738. The vacuum in clinical teaching which resulted led to more students seeking an education in Scotland. Secondly, non-conformist students were denied access to Oxford University, Cambridge University, and Trinity College Dublin. This regulation also resulted in students travelling to Scotland.

Finally, uniquely, a forward-looking Edinburgh Town Council, owned the new medical school, which was founded in 1726. One of the members of the council,

DOI: 10.1201/9781003748816-8

George Drummond, was instrumental in ensuring the quality of the medical school's teaching staff. One of the most significant of these was William Cullen (1710 to 1790), who had a European reputation and was one of the most distinguished physicians of his day. He is remembered for his contributions to technical clinical teaching and for his insistence that patients should be treated as individuals [5]. One of his students was a distinguished surgeon who wrote a textbook of surgery. His name was James Latta, and he expressed his gratitude to Cullen in the advertisement at the beginning of the first volume of his work [6].

INTRODUCTION

James Latta is the earliest of the four Scottish surgeons mentioned above. All three wrote multiple-volume texts on surgery. It has not been possible to find any biographical data on Latta, so all the information about him must be observed or extracted from his texts.

Pain of Surgery and Fear and Post-Operative Comments

Latta had numerous comments on the effects of patient anxieties affecting treatment. He also described characteristics of pain and its management, which could provide information persuading the patient to have the most useful treatment. Fear of the knife was a major patient concern, leading to a demand for the use of a caustic to open a ripe abscess. Latta pointed out that the use of caustics might not be so frightening as a scalpel, but the pain they produce lasted longer than that of the knife, and the spread of the caustic could not be efficiently controlled, so the extent of the painful region could not be controlled. The pain from the knife was indeed sharper, but it was over in an instant, making the knife the preferable implement [7]. He also quoted the experience of other sufferers when informing patients of what they could expect. In one such instance, a patient had delayed surgery for a hernia because she was scared of the pain. Three years after a successful operation, she stated that if she suffered a recurrence, she would not delay an operation because the pain of the disease was much worse than the pain of surgery [8]. Another patient who was operated on for a bladder stone stated after surgery that if he had a recurrence of symptoms, he would call Latta the next day for immediate surgery, as the pain of the operation was so slight compared with the pain of the disease [9].

Pain of Surgery and Anxiety

Latta indicated his awareness of and understanding of the effects of fear on surgical results, which expressed itself in a variety of ways. A fifty-four-year-old man was operated on for a hydrocele. The surgery was expeditious and without problems of any kind, yet the patient died. It turned out that he had hidden the fact that he was so terrified of the prospective operation that he had not slept for the six nights preceding the procedure. After the operation, his pulse rose to 120 and continued to rise until he died [10]. Latta also mentioned the fear of some patients of the incision of peritonsillar abscesses. To cope with this problem, he hid the lancet inside a tube to avoid causing anxiety. This is the same principle as mentioned by Dionis with contempt (see Chapter 7) but is here described as routine. Elsewhere, he commented on the delay in the treatment of breast cancers.

> *It is always to be observed, that the sooner the operation is performed, so much the better; for, if through the negligence or timidity, either of the surgeon or patient, we allow the gland to inflame and ulcerate, there is much less probability of a cure being effected by amputation than in the former cafe [11].*

Opium for Pain Due to Disease or Following Surgery

In a number of situations, Latta proposed giving opium to patients in extreme pain. Indications included pain following nerve injury during bloodletting [12]. Extreme pain from abscesses or gangrene could also require opium. It was further found justified for the quite long period of two months, in what reads like an attack of gout in the left elbow [13]. It was also prescribed for a patient with an incarcerated hernia [14]. Opium with rhubarb was prescribed for tenesmus (Tenesmus is the feeling of the need to pass stools even when the bowel is empty) associated with a fistula in ano. It was also effective in the treatment of an intolerable toothache [15]. Latta also used two grains of opium morning and evening for a syphilitic osteitis (osteitis is inflammation of bone) of the left forearm [16]. The pains were 'somewhat alleviated' in Latta's words. This is reminiscent of a syphilitic osteitis seen by this author during training. Morphine had a limited effect. On the other hand, a single dose of penicillin (unavailable to Latta, obviously) made the patient entirely pain-free and requiring no more morphine. Latta also used opium in some patients who had pain related to trauma. He applied it in ointments as well as prescribing it orally in patients with inflammation or suppuration related post-traumatic pain [17]. It was also of use in controlling the pain of liver abscesses [18]. All of these are indications for the pain of disease, not the pain of surgery. In this respect, Latta continued with the traditional viewpoint. He explained the use of opium to reduce operation pain with the following remark:

> *Opium would perfectly answer the first intention (to reduce patient sensibility), were not its effects upon the system to be dreaded. Large doses of this medicine are very apt to bring on sickness and vomiting, which, after some operations, are much to be dreaded; and therefore its use is laid aside by the most judicious practitioners [19].*

There is no precise information about doses, but there is a significant remark that it should be given in higher doses than had been customary [8, 12]. However, George Young, an Edinburgh physician/surgeon who was a member of the Rankenian Club, which was much involved with the Scottish Enlightenment, had written a treatise on opium. In the introduction, Young stated:

> *Another considerable source of the mischiefs done by this drug, is, the commonly received notion, that opium should be given at any time, when watching or pain is excessive; I am so much of the contrary opinion, that, with me, it is almost a rule not to give it when either of the two is immoderate, e. g. I never give it in obstinate deliriums, a phrenitis, pleuritis, violent gouts, rheumatism, or great inflammations of any kind [20].*

Nonetheless, Latta specified that he had used opium in the treatment of a patient with gout of the elbow for close to two months [13]. The patient came to no harm.

Pain of Surgery and Adjustments of Technique

More than any previous surgeon, Latta outlined modifications of operative technique to minimize the pain patients suffered. For the relatively minor operation of lancing a quinsy, he used a fine spear-pointed lancet, which caused little pain and was preferred to any other instrument [21]. For the major procedure of amputation, he advocated the use of a tourniquet, which made the agonizing cauterization of blood vessels unnecessary. This was yet another repetition of Paré's teaching, mentioned in Chapter 6. The most effective tourniquet had been introduced by Jean-Louis Petit, in Paris. It included a screw mechanism, which made tightening and releasing it much more precise [22]. Finally, the surgeon had to be technically gifted, because dexterity and speed minimized pain, both during lithotomy [9] and amputation [23].

Latta also offered advice concerning the management of trauma. In cases of bullet wounds, management varied according to the depth to which the bullet had penetrated. Also, the material of the bullet had an impact on treatment. Lead balls that had penetrated deeply could be left alone, as experience had shown this was usually safe. However, iron or brass balls should be removed as far as possible because they rusted giving rise to complications. In addition, any accessible cloth forced into the wound should be removed for the same reasons. In superficial wounds, all extraneous material should be removed. Latta emphasized the point that all surgery should be done at the first operation as patients would seldom permit another painful procedure.

Latta was also much concerned with the pain associated with surgery of the nose and mouth. Nasal polyps had traditionally been removed by being pulled out with a forceps or by having their base encircled by a ligature, which was tightened over the following day. This was much less painful [24]. He had a similar attitude to tonsillectomy. Cautery was out of the question because of the risk of damage to normal tissue. Surgical excision carried too great a risk of dangerous haemorrhage. A ligature made of silver wire or catgut was applied to the root of the tonsil and gradually tightened. The tonsil would drop off in a matter of a few days. If both tonsils are swollen, operation on the second side should be delayed until the pain and inflammation following the first operation had settled down. Latta, wishing as always to avoid unnecessary pain, made two extra comments. If the second tonsil did not interfere with breathing and swallowing, it need not be removed. A variation of the ligature treatment introduced by Cheselden would certainly work, but should be avoided, because it included no practical advantage and was associated with extra pain [25]. With tooth extraction, grasp the tooth close to the bone, assuring a good contact with the tooth, then pulling away from the socket and twisting the instrument. This method gave the patient less pain [15].

Latta described two details of abdominal paracentesis which reduced associated discomfort. The location of the abdominal perforation was between the umbilicus and the left iliac spine. The abdomen should be fitted with a belt, which could be tightened as the fluid left the abdomen. Failure to do so led to unpleasant and possibly dangerous symptoms. If these arose, the drainage should be stopped for a while until the symptoms were over. The cross-section of the trocar had evolved through a variety of shapes. The best was an instrument with a sharp-pointed trocar and a circular cross-section. The method described was associated with very little pain.

For anal fistulas, Latta mentioned a procedure of ligation. A flexible silver thread was passed down the fistula to its internal opening. It was then pulled out of the anus, and the two ends were twisted together. This treatment was used by those who feared massive haemorrhage from haemorrhoidal arteries and veins. Latta rejected it because he denied the danger of major bleeding and because such a ligature would be so painful [8].

Finally, Latta has commented on the surgery of the eye. He instructed that if small metallic particles stick upon the cornea, the least painful way to remove them-was with a quill shaped liked a toothpick, moved gently back and forth until the fragment was loosened [26]. If eyelashes scrape on the eyeball, this could be cured by pulling them out with a forceps, though this was painful. A less painful method-was to turn the hairs upwards with a probe and keep them in place for a while with adhesive plaster [27]. Cataracts could be treated by couching or extraction. Latta absolutely preferred couching because it was less painful [28]. In conclusion, he discussed lachrymal fistulae. This is a condition where tears stream down the face when the lachrymal duct between the inner corner of the eye is blocked. In some cases, the blockage could be moved by pressing fluid down the tube with a syringe. However, if this does not work, the canal could be probed. Latta opposed this method of treatment for two reasons. Firstly, the fine probe was incapable of being rigid enough to move a block. More importantly, the treatment was not only ineffective but also very painful [29].

There is no section in Latta's text devoted to the principles of theory and technique on which surgical success was based. He seemed to take it as self-evident that it is more difficult to operate on an object in motion than on one that is still. However, while he did not state the principle as such, more than any previous author, Latta was at pains to describe the need for immobilization in different procedures, often with quite an abundance of detail. The procedures he described where adequate immobilization was needed were aneurysms, hernias, castration, lithotomy, fistula in ano, paraumbilical steatoma, trepanation, eye surgery, nasal polyps, hare lips, cleaning teeth, extracting teeth, thigh amputation, hip-joint amputation, shoulder-joint amputation, and below knee amputation for excision of gangrene. He was a surgeon, who as far as possible left nothing to doubt.

Pain of Cautery

Latta had much to say about cautery, most of it negative. He starts with remarks about the use of actual cautery for removing necrotic bone or caries as it is called. He wrote:

> *The application of the actual cautery must be looked upon as equally inefficacious and injurious; for, if this be applied in such a manner as to destroy entirely the diseased part of the bone, the heat must necessarily destroy also some part of that which was sound, and thus bring on a new caries. If applied in such a manner as not do this, it cannot be supposed to be of any avail [13].*

He thought that actual cautery down to the bone, to close a hernia sac and prevent recurrence, was in fact ineffective [14]. He considered the use of cautery in the treatment of hydroceles to be absurd [30]. Cautery for lachrymal fistula had no advantage over other treatment methods and was to be avoided because it was painful [29]. In one situation, Latta admitted that actual cautery could play a role. This was in cases of cancer of the tongue, which required total removal of the tongue. Referring to the difficulties of haemostasis in this operation he wrote:

> *Yet, notwithstanding this difficulty, we may certainly apply the ligature to some of them, while the blood may be stopped in others, by means of sponge, agaric, or even the actual cautery; for this last terrible remedy seems more admissible here than in any other case whatever [31].*

He objected to the use of actual cautery in cases of caries with severe pain. There were two reasons. It was technically difficult and unreliable. The pain was 'by no means' inferior to that of extracting the tooth [15]. In general, he disliked the use of caustics with one exception, which he described as a cancerous wart on the face. He used caustics, and in the end the lesion was extirpated but at the price of dreadful pain.

Thus, in brief, Latta considered cautery barbaric and tried wherever possible to avoid its use. He specifically stated, in a passage on amputation, that the use of cautery for such operations in the past was dangerous and associated with death [23].

Phlebotomy

In bloodletting, nervous patients were encouraged to lie down, whereas the usual position for the procedure was sitting. A small lancet should be used, as the larger blades made bigger, more painful incisions. Latta recommended careful puncture of veins and avoidance of passing through a vein to perforate its opposite side, which could facilitate perforation of nerves and produce long-lasting pain. It should be avoided and was characterized unequivocally as 'mismanagement' [12]

Diminishing the Pain in Chirurgical Operations [19]

Latta, unlike any predecessor, has written specifically about the pain of surgery in a separate section of his text. What he wrote makes good sense. He describes the methods of making an operation more tolerable:

> *There are two general ways in which this seems possible; one is, by diminishing the sensibility of the patient, so that he may not be capable of feeling very acute pain; the other, by compressing the nerve which goes to the part to be operated upon, so that it cannot feel pain so acutely as it would otherwise do. Opium would perfectly answer the first intention, were not its effects upon the system to be dreaded. Large doses of this medicine are very apt to bring on sickness and vomiting, which, after some operations, are much to be dreaded; and therefore its use is laid aside by the most judicious practitioners [19].*

This has been the standard practice since at least the time of Galen.

Latta then proceeded to mention the work of Mr James Moore, who had described a method for making nerves insensible by compressing them. Since Benjamin Bell had a similar chapter about the pain of surgery and nerve compression, to avoid repetition, the discussion of the topic will be found in a subsequent chapter.

CONCLUSION

From his writings, Latta would appear to have been a humane man and an obsessive surgical technician. He wrote detailed instructions to ensure that patient immobilization was as effective as possible. He decried the use of cautery because of the poor efficacy and dreadful pain associated with its use. He wrote sensibly about the pain of surgery, providing evidence that it could be less than the pain of the disease, which would be useful to tell patients who were dithering about accepting an operation because of anxiety. He also provided evidence of the risks involved in putting anxiety into the driving seat.

Latta used opium for the pain of a variety of diseases and advised high doses and persistence when the clinical situation demanded it. He also gave it to patients after operations. One of the most impressive components of his writing was his readiness to adjust his operative technique to minimize the pain of a procedure. He also mentioned attempts to reduce the pain of amputations by nerve compression, as recommended by Paré and Heister.

Finally, it is deplorable that Latta and his textbooks have not received more attention. They are unusually clearly expressed and, on the basis of their content, represent the work of a major surgical talent. It seems fair to state that James Latta did everything in his power to minimize patient suffering.

REFERENCES

1. Graham HG. *The Social Life of Scotland in the Eighteenth Century*. London: Adams and Charles; 1964.
2. Hamilton D. The Rise of the Professional: 18th Century. In *The Healers: A History of Medicine in Scotland*. Gretna: Firebird Press; 1981.
3. Sutherland S. *Scottish Enlightenment 2013*. Available from: https://www.britannica.com/event/Scottish-Enlightenment/Legacy
4. Macintyre IMC. Enlightenment and Science. Scottish Medicine c1750 - c1850. In: Dingwall H, Hamilton D, Macintyre I, McCrae M, Wright D, editors. *Scottish Medicine and Illustrated History*. Edinburgh: Birlinn Ltd; 2011, pp. 91–151.
5. Cullen W. *Dictionary of Medical Biography*. London: Greenwood Press; 2007, pp. 381–5.
6. Latta J. Advertisement. In *A Practical System of Surgery*. Edinburgh: G Mudie & Son; 1795, pp. 1–2.
7. Latta J. Of the Opening of Abscesses. In *A Practical System of Surgery. I*. Edinburgh: G Mudie & Son; 1795, pp. 31–50.
8. Latta J. Of Fistula in Ano. In *A Practical System of Surgery. II*. Edinburgh: G Mudie & Son; 1795, pp. 39–81.
9. Latta J. Of the Stone in the Bladder. In *A Practical System of Surgery. I*. Edinburgh: G Mudie & Son; 1795, pp. 411–505.

10. Latta J. Hydrocele of the Tunica Vaginalis. In *A Practical System of Surgery. I.* Edinburgh: G Mudie & Son; 1795, pp. 309–73.
11. Latta J. Of Cancerous Breasts. In *A Practical System of Surgery. II.* Edinburgh: G Mudie & Son; 1795, pp. 509–15.
12. Latta J. Of Bloodletting. In *A Practical System of Surgery. I.* Edinburgh: G Mudie & Son; 1795, pp. 5–31.
13. Latta J. Of Inflammation. In *A Practical System of Surgery. I.* Edinburgh: G Mudie & Son; 1795, pp. 88–195.
14. Latta J. Of Herniæ. In *A Practical System of Surgery. I.* Edinburgh: G Mudie & Son; 1795, pp. 196–297.
15. Latta J. Of the Toothache. In *A Practical System of Surgery. II.* Edinburgh: G Mudie & Son; 1795, pp. 407–23.
16. Latta J. Of Simple Exostosis, and of Venereal Exostoses, or Nodes. In *A Practical System of Surgery. II.* Edinburgh: G Mudie & Son; 1795, pp. 517–26.
17. Latta J. Of Wounds in General. In *A Practical System of Surgery. III.* Edinburgh: G Mudie & Son; 1795, pp. 1–88.
18. Latta J. Inflammation and Abscess of the Liver. In *A Practical System of Surgery. III.* Edinburgh: G Mudie & Son; 1795, pp. 271–8.
19. Latta J. Of Diminishing the Pain of Chirurgical Operations. In *A Practical System of Surgery. II.* Edinburgh: G Mudie & Son; 1795, pp. 533–4.
20. Young G. The Preface. In *A Treatise on Opium.* London: A. Millar; 1753, pp. iii–x.
21. Latta J. Angina and Quinsey. In *A Practical System of Surgery. III.* Edinburgh: G Mudie & Son; 1795, pp. 268–71.
22. Kirkup J. The Mechanical Arrest of Hemorrhage. In *The Evolution of Surgical Instruments.* Novato, CA: historyofscience.com; 2006, pp. 311–32.
23. Latta J. Of the Method of Performing Amputation. In *A Practical System of Surgery. III.* Edinburgh: G Mudie & Son; 1795, pp. 586–92.
24. Latta J. Of the Polypus of the Nose. In *A Practical System of Surgery. II.* Edinburgh: G Mudie & Son; 1795, pp. 305–17.
25. Latta J. Of the Enlargement and Extirpation of Tonsils. In *A Practical System of Surgery. II.* Edinburgh: G Mudie & Son; 1795, pp. 318–22.
26. Latta J. Of Ophthalmia, or Inflammation of the Eyes. In *A Practical System of Surgery. II.* Edinburgh: G Mudie & Son; 1795, pp. 184–92.
27. Latta J. Of the Inchiasis, or Inversion of the Cilia. In *A Practical System of Surgery. II.* Edinburgh: G Mudie & Son; 1795, pp. 208–14.
28. Latta J. Of Extracting the Cataract. In *A Practical System of Surgery. II.* Edinburgh: G Mudie & Son; 1795, pp. 263–79.
29. Latta J. *Of the Fistula Lachrymalis.* In *A Practical System of Surgery. II.* Edinburgh: G Mudie & Son; 1795, pp. 279–301.
30. Latta J. Of the Hydrocele. In *A Practical System of Surgery. I.* Edinburgh: G Mudie & Son; 1795, pp. 297–373.
31. Latta J. Of Ulcers in the Mouth and Tongue, and Extirpation of Part of the Tongue Itself. In *A Practical System of Surgery. II.* Edinburgh: G Mudie & Son; 1795, pp. 357–64.

9 Surgical Pain – Transition to the Nineteenth Century: Benjamin Bell (1749–1806)

INTRODUCTION

Benjamin Bell was born in April 1749 in Dumfries to a family that had owned estates in the neighbourhood since the fifteenth century. His father was George Bell, and his mother was Anne née Corrie. His father was a successful farmer but, on occasion, exhibited a tendency to play frivolous pranks and also to a certain small-mindedness. His mother was calm, placid, and pious. It may be noted that George Bell died in 1813 and his wife some years later, so that both Benjamin Bell's parents survived him [1].

Bell received his early training from James Hill, a distinguished Dumfries surgeon [2]. While regrettably forgotten in later times, he was a much-respected practitioner in his day [2, 3]. From the project 'Eighteenth century medics' there is a record of Hill who trained altogether over twenty young surgeons all of whom paid between £1 and £45. He started the training of Benjamin Bell in 1764, but no fee was charged [4]. The reason for this is not stated, but Bell's grandfather was a landowner, and his father was a well-to-do farmer, and it is easy to believe that his family and Hill's moved in the same social circles with Bell's family having the edge socially, since the publicly distinguished member of Hill's family was his wife [3]. Bell's training with Hill started in 1764, when he was only fifteen years old. Two years later, when he was seventeen, he proceeded to the Edinburgh medical school, which had grown to great prominence and was respected throughout Europe. Bell settled in Edinburgh and was admitted a Fellow of the Royal College of Surgeons on 5 April 1771 at the tender age of twenty-two. His 'System of Surgery' was first published in 1783. It ran to many editions. It included seven volumes, partly due to the range of topics and partly due to Bell's discursive style of writing. Evidence for this statement may be seen by comparing the number of pages used for the topic of bloodletting, Latta uses twenty-seven and Bell uses ninety-two. Bell's writing style is also unconventional in one other aspect, being the second surgeon in this book to present his material using the first-person singular. It should be noted that, since Bell's mammoth work was published in multiple editions, the organization of material between editions varied. For this reason, all the volumes used for reference in this book are part of the same edition, the sixth from 1796. All volumes could not be found for any other edition.

DOI: 10.1201/9781003748816-9

Pain of Surgery

Bell has some comments to make on how to convince patients of the best course of action. One example concerns poisoned wounds. The aim of treatment is removal of the affected region. The available treatments were excision with the knife or the cautery or application of caustics including an ointment containing mercury. In a rather muddled passage, it would seem Bell tried to persuade patients that the brief pain of the knife or cautery was preferrable to the long-lasting pain of a caustic ointment stating:

> *...a timid patient may indeed hesitate in the use of such a formidable remedy, when he knows that we are possessed of an antidote which seldom fails. Many, however, would endure the momentary pain of a burn or a cut, in preference to the slow operation of a mercurial course [5].*

Bell commented on avoiding pain in many locations all over the body. If inspection of the cranium was required, a linear incision gave just as good exposure as the conventional cruciate and T-shaped incisions, took much less time, and healed more easily [6]. Like Latta, he considered a ligature the best treatment for nasal polyps. Excision with a scalpel was impractical because the root of the polyps lay deep inside the nasal passage. Cautery was inappropriate because the local anatomy made it impossible to remove the pathological tissue without injuring normal adjacent tissue. This left extraction by tearing it with forceps. The ligature was more effective and much less painful, and was therefore to be preferred [7]. The ligature was also preferred for tonsillectomy (removing tonsils) since excision carried a risk of severe haemorrhage, and cauterization, whether actual or potential, would damage surrounding normal tissue [8]. Toothache was common, and Bell noted that care should be taken to avoid gum injury during tooth extraction, as so doing materially reduced the pain of the procedure [9].

Bell also had a comment on unavoidable severe pain from life-saving surgery. Of extirpation of the eye, he writes:

> *...the extirpation of an eye, is attended with much pain to the patient, and appears to be of a cruel and dangerous nature to bye-standers; so that few surgeons have resolution to perform it. It ought in no instance to be advised where a cure can be accomplished by means of a more gentle nature; but when this cannot be done, and when a patient will for certain die in misery if the eye be not removed, it ought surely to be recommended as a means that may afford at least some chance of safety. For although it will not always prove successful, yet we know from experience, that in some instances lives have been saved by means of it, which otherwise would, probably have been lost [10].*

Bell described a considerable number of instances where the operative technique was adjusted to minimize pain. Suppurating venereal inguinal lymph glands were called buboes from the Greek 'βουβών', which means groin. Once suppuration was ripe, the swelling should be opened. Since this was very painful, the incision into the capsule should be large enough to drain effectively thereby avoiding a second painful procedure [11]. During orchiectomy (removal of a testis), care must be taken not to include nerves in the spermatic cord in a ligature [12]. Bell also invented a special instrument for the treatment of phimosis (Phimosis is a condition where the foreskin is too tight to be pulled back from the head of the penis) [13]. In addition, he decried the use of ligatures for the treatment of anal fistulae as more painful than other treatment methods, and therefore not justified because it was not more effective [14].

Wounds should be examined for foreign material, which should be removed. However, this should be done gently, to avoid pain. Moreover, if the wound was deep, enthusiasm for the thorough removal of foreign material was misplaced. It was possible for buried foreign material to remain in the body without causing any inconvenience. However, like Latta he specified that the nature of the foreign material was important, since lead was tolerated, whereas wood, glass, iron, or cloth were more dangerous [15]. When examining thoracic wounds, a fairly large blunt bougie prevented penetrating too far and was also less painful than a narrower instrument [16]. If there was tension in ligatures used to close the abdomen, and the patient complained of pain, the ligatures should be loosened [17]. Removing deep penetrating bullets might be easier from the opposite side, rather than operating down the path the bullet had taken. The pain of incising the skin directly over a bullet was less than that produced by tearing it out of a deep wound with forceps [18].

Bell noted that covering bare areas because of skin excision during surgery required a long and painful post-operative course. Mastectomy for breast cancer was a case in point. It had been traditional to remove all the skin covering morbid tissue underneath. Retaining as much skin as possible simplified post-operative care and spared the patient much distress [19].

Bell also described the techniques of immobilization necessary for successful surgery. These included eye surgery, dental extraction, tracheotomy, mastectomy, hernia surgery, hydrocele surgery, testicle extirpation, bladder punctures, thigh amputation, shoulder amputation, and Caesarean section.

Like Latta, Bell has a brief chapter concerned with reducing the pain of surgery, including the mention of Mr James Moore's device for compressing nerves [20]. This will be considered in a subsequent chapter. From the above text it must be clear that Bell consistently exercised himself to the benefit of his patients not least in his efforts to minimize the pain of surgery.

Pain of Cautery

Pain from cautery is a minor component of Bell's writing as he provided multiple instances where it was inapplicable or inferior. Caustics used to open an abscess with the ensuing diffusion into adjacent normal tissue made it an inferior technique compared to the scalpel [21]. It was also mentioned that actual cautery had been tried in cases of Goitre but had not been found beneficial [22].

Bell was in favour of using cautery to remove the tissue around poisoned wounds, such as those inflicted by rabid dogs. On the whole, patients preferred the momentary pain of a cut or a burn to the prolonged pain of a caustic [5]. On the other hand, in the case of bone caries, Bell was of the opinion that cautery did more harm than good.

The aim of actual cautery for toothache was to destroy the relevant nerve. However, in most cases it could not be performed deep enough to be effective, because the pain was intolerable [9]. However, it is admitted that if there is serious haemorrhage as a complication of oral surgery, actual cautery may be needed [23]. Cauterizing a location behind the ear to treat toothache was abandoned as ineffective not least because the treatment is more painful than a tooth extraction [24]. Cautery in the treatment of hernias was simply unreliable [25]. Using a caustic to remove a diseased testis was far too painful, and the pain lasted much longer than excision with a knife [12]. Cautery should never be used in the removal of haemorrhoids, because ligature was so much simpler and less painful [26]. Perianal warts should be removed with the knife, as there was no risk of haemorrhage. However, if the patient was too nervous, caustics might be used. But, it was important to ensure that the caustic did not reach the gut, which could produce complications [27].

Analgesics

George Young was an Edinburgh surgeon and actively involved in the Scottish Enlightenment. Bell most probably was aware of George Young's monograph on the use of opium. Young died in 1757 when Bell was only eight years old. On the other hand, Young had been mentor to James Hill who had been Bell's first teacher in surgery. There seems little doubt that Bell had a profound belief in the usefulness of the drug. What follows, concerns opium taken orally. One principle, in keeping with the teachings of Latta was that it should be given in adequate doses, judged by the pain relief obtained [28].

Bell advocated its use in a number of inflammations. These include phlegmons (diffuse areas of inflammation) [29]. It was also valuable in the management of abscesses, for example in breast abscesses in women [30] or lymph node abscesses arising from venereal disease [11]. It was also useful in cases of spina ventosa when there was severe pain. (Spina ventosa is an outdated term for a cystic enlargement of bones, which is now known to be a form of tuberculosis) [31]. Finally, with regard to inflammation there was a condition Bell refers to as a 'vitiated ulcer', the pain of which benefitted from opium. This was an ulcer where the appearances of the matter produced differed from that of a purulent ulcer. Such matter was thin green, acrid, and included gelatinous elements [32]. Finally, with burns, the dose of opium should be adjusted so as to relieve the pain [33].

Opium was also useful for pain in victims of trauma. The best preparation for pain from simple incised wounds was taken orally and applied topically, preferably in multiple small doses [15]. In post-traumatic gangrene it was useful [34]. For the pain in injured joints, opium was the only effective medication [35]. Thoracic wounds could require large doses of opium [36] as could gunshot wounds [18]. It was also useful following injury to the eye [37]. Bell also advocated the use of opium cranial injury for pain associated with cerebral concussion [38], cranial contusion [39] and meningeal inflammation [40]. This would not be considered advisable today but was sensible at the time it was recommended.

There is some mention of the use of opium in the context of vascular pathology. If pain followed bloodletting, it was useful [41]. It was also helpful prior to surgery and during the post-operative phase of surgery for aneurysms [42]. Opiates were also valuable in eye disease either in the early stages of an eye abscess [37] or before extirpation of an eye for cancer [10].

Pains related to teeth were also treated with opium, including teething. Most general practitioners know that the most important reason for treating the pain of teething is to enable the mothers to sleep, because the crying night after night for perhaps months can be extremely enervating. To those of us who have prescribed paracetamol and orange juice for this condition, the idea that opium could be used while inappropriate is not without its attraction. Thus, Bell's use of it for this purpose reflects a small taste of the advantages of ignorance [43]. Laudanum, which is a solution of opium in alcohol, was prescribed for toothache with gum swelling [44].

Finally, opium was useful in the management of hernias both before surgery [25] and as a post-operative analgesic [45]. With hydroceles, opium was useful in the event gangrene developed [46] or in cases where the testis became inflamed [47]. Opium was also used in cases of bladder stone, both prior to surgery and also as a post-operative analgesic [48].

Phlebotomy

Bloodletting was considered a minor procedure, but it could give rise to problems. A small knife blade was superior. With larger blades, the skin incision was bigger than the incision in the vein, thus producing unnecessary pain without any practical advantage. The lancet should enter the vein obliquely and only open the outer surface of a vein [29]. If the inner surface was also penetrated, there was the risk of damaging an adjacent nerve producing pain. This pain was entirely the fault of the operator and should be avoided [49]. A similar complication could occur following the inclusion of a nerve within an arterial ligature [41].

CONCLUSION

The text a surgeon writes does not only provide information about the topics under advisement but also can reveal aspects of the writer's personality. Careful reading of such medieval surgeons as Theodoric or Henri de Mondeville is revealing. Theodoric makes arrogant-sounding remarks, though this may not be surprising because he was not only a surgeon but also a bishop and the personal physician to a pope. Henri de Mondeville, writing about optimal surgical technique, made statements about his predecessors which are simply untrue but which supported arguments he wished to make [50]. Daniel Turner at a young age saw fit to publish material that was critical of some practitioners. He was motivated by passion and very probably the awareness of his own considerable talent. It did not, however, help his career [51].

Benjamin Bell did not engage in such polemics. There can be little doubt he was a kindly man who worked very hard and did his best to minimize the pain of treatment. Examples of this are the recommendation to use a narrow lancet for bloodletting and his opposition to all forms of cautery unless unavoidable. He had far more mentions of opium in his text than any earlier surgeon. However, no matter how well meaning Bell was, there remains a difficulty related to the clarity of his writing. A most distinguished English surgeon and scientist, Sir Benjamin Brodie wrote:

> *During the following summer (1802), I passed my time much as I had done formerly. I thought, however, that I ought to do something towards advancing my professional knowledge, and, accordingly, I borrowed Benjamin Bell's 'System of Surgery' from Mr. Wyche, one of the surgeons to the Salisbury Infirmary. I found it, however, a most unreadable production; indeed, I doubt whether it was ever read by any one. Yet, somehow, it had a sort of reputation in its day, which, I imagine, is to be attributed to it being the work of a leading surgeon in Edinburgh, and to its consisting: of some half-dozen thick octavo volumes [52].*

While harsh, extensive reading of Bell's books has led this author to understand exactly what Brodie meant. Bell's writing is full of examples of his kindness and consideration. Unfortunately, the lack of clarity can make it difficult to understand precisely what he meant.

REFERENCES

1. Bell B. His Progenitors-His Father, George Bell. In *The Life and Character & Writings of Benjamin Bell, by His Grandson Benjamin Bell*. Edinburgh: Edmonston and Douglas; 1868, pp. 1–10.
2. Hill J. *Oxford Dictionary of National Biography*. Oxford: Oxford University Press; 2006, pp. 1–3.
3. Ganz JC. *James Hill - a Dumfries Neurosurgeon*. Newcastle upon Tyne: Cambridge Scholars Publishing; 2022.
4. Wallis PJ, Wallis RV, Whittet TD, Burnby JGL. *Eighteenth Century Medics (Subscriptions, Licences, Apprencticeships)*. Newcastle upon Tyne: Project for Historical Biobigliography; 1985.
5. Bell B. Of Poisoned Wounds. In *A System of Surgery. II*. 6th ed. Edinburgh: Bell & Bradfute; 1796, pp. 163–75.
6. Bell B. Of Compression of the Brain, from Fractures attended with Depression of teh Skull. In *A System of Surgery. III*. 6th ed. Edinburgh: Bell & Bradfute; 1796, pp. 265–337.
7. Bell B. Of Polypi in the Nose and Throat. In *A System of Surgery. IV*. 6th ed. Edinburgh: Bell & Bradfute; 1796, pp. 394–436.
8. Bell B. Of Extirpation of Tonsils. In *A System of Surgerey. IV*. 6th ed. Edinburgh: Bell & Bradfute; 1796, pp. 437–46.
9. Bell B. Of Toothach from the Nerve being Laid Bare, and of the Various Methods of Extracting Teeth. In *A System of Surgery. V*. 6th ed. Edinburgh: Bell & Bradfute; 1796, pp. 11–63.
10. Bell B. Of Cancer of the Eye, and Extirpation of the Eye-ball. In *A System of Surgery. IV*. 6th ed. Edinburgh: Bell & Bradfute; 1796, pp. 171–80.
11. Bell B. Of Venereal Buboes. In *A System of Surgery. I*. 6th ed. Edinburgh: Bell & Bradfute; 1796, pp. 152–66.
12. Bell B. Of the Sarcocele, or Schirrous Testicle. In *A System of Surgery. VI*. 6th ed. Edinburgh: Bell & Bradfute; 1796, pp. 16–56.
13. Bell B. Of the Phymosis. In *A System of Surgery. VI*. 6th ed. Edinburgh: Bell & Bradfute; 1796, pp. 57–64.

14. Bell B. Of the Fistula in Ano. In *A System of Surgery. VI.* 6th ed. Edinburgh: Bell & Bradfute; 1796, pp. 365–417.
15. Bell B. Of the Cure of Simple Incised Wounds. In *A System of Surgery. I.* 6th ed. Edinburgh: Bell & Bradfute; 1796, pp. 357–423.
16. Bell B. Of General Remarks on Wounds of the Thorax. In *A System of Surgery. II.* 6th ed. Edinburgh: Bell & Bradfute; 1796, pp. 33–48.
17. Bell B. Of Wounds that Penetrate the Cavity of the Abdomen, but Which do not Injure Any of the CONTAINED PARTS. In *A System of Surgery. II.* 6th ed. Edinburgh: Bell & Bradfute; 1796, pp. 101–24.
18. Bell B. Of Gunshot Wounds. In *A System of Surgery. II.* 6th ed. Edinburgh: Bell & Bradfute; 1796, pp. 176–206.
19. Bell B. Of the Amputation of Cancerous Mammæ. In *A System of Surgery. V.* 6th ed. Edinburgh: Bell & Bradfute; 1796, pp. 169–90.
20. Bell B. Of Preventing or Diminishing Pain in Chirurgical Operations. In *A System of Surgery. VII.* 6th ed. Edinburgh: Bell & Bradfute; 1796, pp. 393–7.
21. Bell B. Of the different Methods of Opening Abscesses. In *A System of Surgery. 1.* 6th ed. Edinburgh: Bell & Bradfute; 1796, pp. 72–87.
22. Bell B. Of Bronchocele. In *A System of Surgery. 1.* 6th ed. Edinburgh: Bell & Bradfute; 1796, pp. 283–97.
23. Bell B. Of Ulcers of the Mouth and Tongue and Extirpation of the Tongue. In *A System of Surgery.V.* 6th ed. Edinburgh: Bell & Bradfute; 1796, pp. 91–7.
24. Bell B. Of perforating the Lobes of the Ears. In *A System of Surgery. V.* 6th ed. Edinburgh: Bell & Bradfute; 1796, pp. 125–7.
25. Bell B. Of Herniæ in General. In *A System of Surgery. V.* 6th ed. Edinburgh: Bell & Bradfute; 1796, pp. 255–311.
26. Bell B. Of Hæmorrhoids, or Piles. In *A System of Surgery. VI.* 6th ed. Edinburgh: Bell & Bradfute; 1796, pp. 329–44.
27. Bell B. Of Condylomatous Excrescences, and Similar Affections about the Anus. In *A System of Surgery. VI.* 6th ed. Edinburgh: Bell & Bradfute; 1796, pp. 345–8.
28. Bell B. Of the Ligature of Arteries and other Means Employed by Art for Putting a Stop to Hemorrhagies. In *A System of Surgery. III.* 6th ed. Edinburgh: Bell & Bradfute; 1796, pp. 40–75.
29. Bell B. Remarks on the Preparations of Lead, and Other Sedatives. In *A System of Surgery. I.* 6th ed. Edinburgh: Bell & Bradfute; 1796, pp. 35–49.
30. Bell B. *A System of Surgery*. 6th ed. Edinburgh: Bell & Bradfute; 1796.
31. Bell B. Of Simple Exostosis, Venereal Nodes, and Spina Ventosa. In *A System of Surgery. I.* 6th ed. Edinburgh: Bell & Bradfute; 1796, pp. 310–32.
32. Bell B. Of the Cure of the Simple Vitiated Ulcer. In *A System of Surgery. II.* 6th ed. Edinburgh: Bell & Bradfute; 1796, pp. 297–307.
33. Bell B. Of Burns. In *A System of Surgery. II.* 6th ed. Edinburgh: Bell & Bradfute; 1796, pp. 207–17.
34. Bell B. Of Lacerated and Contused Wounds. In *A System of Surgery. I.* 6th ed. Edinburgh: Bell & Bradfute; 1796, pp. 438–54.
35. Bell B. Of Wounds in the Ligaments. In *A System of Surgery. I.* 6th ed. Edinburgh: Bell & Bradfute; 1796, pp. 474–88.
36. Bell B. Of Wounds of the Diaphragm, Mediastinum, and Pericardium. In *A System of Surgery. II.* 6th ed. Edinburgh: Bell & Bradfute; 1796, pp. 77–83.
37. Bell B. Of Abscesses in the Globe of the Eye. In *A System of Surgery. IV.* 6th ed. Edinburgh: Bell & Bradfute; 1796, pp. 102–13.

38. Bell B. Of Concussion or Commotion of the Brain. In *A System of Surgery III.* 6th ed. Edinburgh: Bell & Bradfute; 1796, pp. 355–68.
39. Bell B. Of Contusion of the Head. In *A System of Surgery. III.* 6th ed. Edinburgh: Bell & Bradfute; 1796, pp. 377–407.
40. Bell B. Conclusion. In *A System of Surgery. III.* 6th ed. Edinburgh: Bell & Bradfute; 1796, pp. 423–32.
41. Bell B. Of Wounds or Pricks in the Nerves and Tendons. In *A System of Surgery. III.* 6th ed. Edinburgh: Bell & Bradfute; 1796, pp. 116–40.
42. Bell B. Of the Treatment of Aneurisms. In *A System of Surgery. III.* 6th ed. Edinburgh: Bell & Bradfute; 1796, pp. 212–37.
43. Bell B. Of Dentition. In *A System of Surgery. IV.* 6th ed. Edinburgh: Bell & Bradfute; 1796, pp. 498–504.
44. Bell B. Of Toothache from Inflammation. In *A System of Surgery. V.* 6th ed. Edinburgh: Bell & Bradfute; 1796, pp. 63–8.
45. Bell B. Of the Bubonocele. In *A System of Surgery. V.* 6th ed. Edinburgh: Bell & Bradfute; 1796, pp. 312–51.
46. Bell B. Of the Anarcous Hydrocele of the Scrotum. In *A System of Surgery. V.*. 6th ed. Edinburgh: Bell & Bradfute; 1796, pp. 393–407.
47. Bell B. Of the Hydrocele of the Tunica Vaginalis Testis. In *A System of Surgery. V.*. 6th ed. Edinburgh: Bell & Bradfute; 1796, pp. 408–507.
48. Bell B. Of the Lateral Operation. In *A System of Surgery. VI.* 6th ed. Edinburgh: Bell & Bradfute; 1796, pp. 148–216.
49. Bell B. Of Wounds in General. In *A System of Surgery. I.* 6th ed. Edinburgh: Bell & Bradfute; 1796, pp. 333–56.
50. Ganz JC. *Laudable Pus. Neurosurgery before Science: Taking A Chance.* Newcastle upon Tyne: Cambridge Scholars Publishing; 2021, pp. 97–126.
51. Turner D. *Apologia Chyrurgica.* London: J. Whitlock; 1695.
52. Hawkins C. Autobiography. In *The Works of Sir Benjamin Collins Brodie.* London: Longman, Green, Longman, Roberts & Green; 1865, pp. 1–116.

10 Surgical Pain – Transition to the Nineteenth Century: John Bell (1763–1820)

INTRODUCTION

John Bell was the second of four brothers, children of Rev. William Bell (1704–1779) and Margaret Morrice. William Bell was ordained into the Presbyterian Church of Scotland but converted to the Episcopal Church [1, 2]. This meant he supported the Stuart Family, which meant he would have supported the unsuccessful 1745 rebellion. His change of conviction led to financial loss, and the Bell children were brought up in straightened circumstances if not exactly poverty. Their mother was a devout and learned woman, and all four boys made impressive careers. Robert, the eldest, became Professor of Conveyancing to the Society of Writers to the Signet. George occupied the Chair of Scots Law in Edinburgh University and was an acknowledged master of commercial jurisprudence. Charles of course became eponymous three times with his law, his long thoracic nerve, and his palsy. A more distinguished medical career would be hard to imagine.

John Bell qualified as a surgeon in 1786 and was admitted as a Freeman Surgeon Apothecary in the new institution of the Royal College and Corporation of Surgeon Apothecaries of Edinburgh. This gave him the right to practice surgery in the Royal Infirmary [2].

Accurate surgery depends on accurate anatomy. At the time, Edinburgh was a leading centre for the study of anatomy, where the second of the three Alexander Monros was professor of Anatomy. It was he who gave his name to the foramen between the lateral ventricles of the brain and the third ventricle. However, he was a physician, and his anatomy teaching was formal and systematic. By contrast, John Bell considered anatomy should be taught in a way that benefited surgeons. In this, he was a notable pioneer, setting up in competition as it were to the Monros; and he was notably successful [2]. He wrote an anatomy of bones, muscles, and joints in 1793. This was followed in 1797 by 'The Anatomy and Physiology of the Human Body'. His books were more valuable because he was a talented artist who could draw realistic illustrations of the anatomy he described. In this, he was at times assisted by his brother Charles, who was an even better artist.

John Bell continued to teach surgery up to 1799 at which point he was barred from practice in the Royal Infirmary, which essentially stopped his teaching career. He concentrated on surgery and became regarded as the leading surgeon in Edinburgh.

DOI: 10.1201/9781003748816-10

The opposition to Bell was led by James Gregory (1753–1821) who was Professor of Medicine and a Manager of the Infirmary. This James Gregory was capable of gross impropriety. On one occasion, he thrashed the gynaecologist James Hamilton (1767–1839) with a cane. For this, he was fined £100 (around £12,000 in 2025). He showed no regret and stated he would happily pay another fine for the pleasure of doing it again [3]. There was then as now discord between physicians and surgeons, but Gregory wrote thus:

Of the many individuals, who in the course of this century are to become Fellows of the Royal College of Surgeons in Edinburgh, some will be half mad, and others more than half stupid; some will be grossly ignorant of their profession, of which perhaps they may never have learned any more than just enough to enable them to pass at their examination; and even this little they may have learned by means of a Short Catechism, which they never understood, but only got by rote...

Some may have excellent fingers and thumbs, but without brains enough to know when and how to use them; others may have brains enough, and these very good of their kind, who may be lamentably deficient in point of fingers and thumbs; some may be savages in their dispositions, and brutes in their manners; some may be very fine gentlemen, minutely acquainted with all the most fashionable cures for the fashionable distemper, and perhaps well qualified to treat any common cafe of that most important disorder, but withal of such general character, habits, and conduct, that no person in his senses would ever think of employing them for the cure of any other disease [4].

This is so offensive that it would seem to be incapable of being accepted, but Bell remained excluded from the Infirmary.

PRINCIPLES OF SURGERY

On the first page of the first volume of his book, Bell presents an important concept. Operations are not the whole of surgery despite the associated drama [5]. They may be considered the least part of the profession's activities. He notes that surgeons can become anxious during surgery but should remember that they are not as anxious as their patients [6]. He further mentions that what the knife cures it must destroy while what the bandage cures is saved [7].

Bell made some interesting remarks about fractures. He is the only surgeon to make realistic remarks about the treatment of fractures at a time when X-rays did not exist to outline the anatomy of a fracture.

Ask a young man who has studied his profession faithfully, what he would do with a fractured limb? he cannot tell. Ask the same question of one who has practised his profession long, who has, moreover, practised it well and sensibly ? He can hardly tell how he himself is accustomed to manage a fractured limb! He has no rule nor settled method! he waits for the particular case, trusts in his own consciousness of sense and experience, and provides for difficulties only after they have come upon him

Degrading as this may appear to our profession, it is, I fear, but too certain, that while more has been written on the subject of fractures than on hernia, lithotomy, amputation, or trepan, yet no two books correspond, no two authors agree, even on the general points of practice; and every surgeon, whether in the army or in the navy, in a village or in a city, sets a broken limb as he writes his name, after a fashion of his own [8].

Bell provided sensible advice for a variety of surgical emergencies, advice which amongst other things would minimize pain. If a patient with head injury were struggling and refused to submit, trepanation was not necessary, a view with which most modern neurosurgeons could agree [9]. He insisted that if it became clear that amputation was unavoidable, persisting with any other long and painful procedure was not justified. In addition, he stated what all surgeons should understand that sometimes doing nothing was the right course of action. [10]. Another piece of wisdom he pronounced, in the context of nasal polyps, was that poor people were hardy and ignored their health and did not present with tumours that were not producing seriously inconvenient symptoms [11]. Finally, in a discussion of the various kinds of lithotomy, he stated a vital principle which seems self-evident yet in the heat of the moment can so easily be forgotten. He insisted that the surgeon may cause pain only if by so doing he is preventing long-term suffering [12].

THE IMPACT OF FEAR ON SURGICAL RESULTS

Fear of surgery is in large measure fear of the expected pain. The one case of John Bell's where a patient's fear led to her death, is a horror story. It emphasizes the dearth of expectations of patients and surgeons in the eighteenth century and earlier times, which should be recalled when trying to assess the judgements and actions of our forefathers. Briefly, a Scottish woman in her middle twenties, living in London, had been struck on the head by a smoothing iron which had been insecurely attached to the wall above her head. There was a portion of the cranium that was detached from the rest, but which resisted extraction on many occasions during the months she lay in hospital. Throughout this period attempts were made to remove the injured bone but without success. Then she retired to the country for three to four months, during which time she improved. However, on returning to hospital she again deteriorated. Finally, she returned to her home in Scotland, but prior to her departure her medical attendants advised her to avoid surgery at all costs. She lay in hospital and refused an operation until she became so weakened that she agreed, albeit with a bad grace. Some infected bone was removed but by no means all. The wound observed at operation was described. The scalp had sloughed off over an area with a diameter of five to six inches. The extent of cranial caries was three by five inches. Much loose bone had mouldered away. The scalp edges were swollen, livid, painful, and pus was profuse, dark, and stinking. It was discharging through the external ear having eroded the roof of the external ear canal. The pus had extended down into the neck where it formed a large collection, but the patient refused drainage. A combination of bad advice and personal anxiety undoubtedly resulted in the death of the young lady.

This is very unfamiliar for a neurosurgeon in the twenty-first century. The professional literature on the topic of caries is very limited, with only one reference to a case study in the Journal of Neurosurgery [13], and a few references mentioned in that paper and a book chapter published in the same year. They were all earlier than 1946 [14]. The term caries is not to be found in the index of a well-known textbook of surgery [15]. Yet it was a familiar term from the seventeenth to the nineteenth century. It was mentioned by Wiseman [16], Paré [17], Turner [18], Heister [19], Le Dran [20], Benjamin Bell [21], and John Bell [22]. It is well to remember that our predecessors were dealing with conditions of which we have no knowledge.

The above case was the only one of Bell's cases in which the anxieties of the patient and her surgeons impacted negatively on the outcome of treatment. He did however comment on the details of patient behaviour which could affect results. He presented this information in relation to social standing. The poor he described as improvident, stubborn, and unable to assess remote consequences. In addition, they were so accustomed to discomfort so that slight pain or deformity was not a worry, when compared with losing work and hence the money needed to support the family. In addition, from whom should they seek advice? Distance from qualified care and lack of funds mitigated against seeking aid.

The rich on the other hand might be timid, and seeking the comfortable advice of the insufficiently qualified delayed accepting the harsh reality associated with, for example, a growing tumour. They believed in the spontaneous cure of tumours, and accepted patent medicines. Finally, the surgeon whose reputation was expanding did not wish to damage it by undertaking a procedure that could damage a patient or even hasten death [10].

PAIN OF SURGERY

Bell provided detailed sensible advice about how the head should be held during trepanation [23]. He also immobilized a patient in the most humane way possible for the operation of lithotomy. This involved three assistants and a large firm steady table covered with a folded blanket. A friend should be present to encourage and support the patient and to supply water and wine when needed [24].

Bell has sensible comments on speed. Dexterity is appropriate to reduce the duration of the patient's suffering. However, it must take second place to safety when the dissection is in critical areas where care is required to avoid inflicting further damage to the patient [5]. He discussed wound healing at length pointing out what delays healing and emphasizing that delayed healing produces pain [25]. The pain of suppurating joints could be relieved with an ointment containing camphor and laudanum [26]. Bell stated one error of fact. He stated that the dura is insensible even to cautery [27]. This is true unless a dural artery is cut and requires diathermy. In my experience, this is quite painful.

Having stated his preference for the knife and the forceps in the treatment of nasal polyps, Bell thought that for the biggest lesions, ligature was to be preferred. Apparently, the first tightening of the ligature loop was very painful, and this was unavoidable [11]. He described operations for complex tumours in the mouth and neck. He repeated the need to slow down a dissection, where separating the tissues from each other is dangerous. He also recalled the application of this principle to specific cases, recording the reactions of the patients. He demonstrated sympathy and concern. The beautiful drawings illustrated just how difficult the surgery must have been. He made a powerful and considered statement about the influence of pain on an operator, which yet again seems to have been influenced by the writings of Celsus.

> *The surgeon, when he speaks of courage, must always distinguish the discreet and deliberate boldness which belong to his professional character, from the personal bravery, or fool-hardy contempt of danger, which he is entitled to indulge in his own individual case; it may to himself seem heroic, or gallant, to endanger, or to throw away life; but,*

> *when responsible for that of a fellow-creature, he has no such latitude of sentiment or action, and must be guided, not by feeling, but reason. So strictly is he bound to avoid danger, that he is actually bound to afflict his patient with protracted and severe pains, to ensure his safety; and to endure the unmerited reproaches of whatever ignorant or ill-judging person may choose to report his operations as awkward or slow. Dispatch and a show of dexterity will ever be a poor apology for endangering life;—and pain, a bad reason for hurry or perturbation, where loss of blood may be the forfeit: the pain of pulling the stump of a corrupted tooth is more severe and often more protracted than that of the most important operations; the pain of simple incisions is never deadly [28].*

PAIN AND CAUTERY

Bell was very much aware of the pain of cautery. He recounted the agonies the technique can inflict when it was used for haemostasis and found no place for it, and indeed deplored its use. Nonetheless, he approved of the use of cauterization to delay the progress of scrofulous disease of the hip (tuberculous arthritis). Otherwise, he avoided the use of the cautery. On the other hand, he retained an interest in the use of caustics. He found them useful in the treatment of ulcers [29]. They also could play a part in operations on nasal polyps, which seem to have given Bell a great deal of trouble [30]. Caustics could also have a part to play with tumours of the throat [31]. Finally, caustics may occasionally be useful in treating the bed of an arteriovenous fistula, where possible remnants of the lesion may be observed [32].

ANALGESICS

In contrast with Benjamin Bell and James Latta, John Bell's books contain few mentions of opium. Moreover, his reasons for using it are somewhat different. He states that it us useful in checking diarrhoea and fever, since these are exacerbated by irritation and pain. Following wounds, the patient may be rigid, shaking, cold, and tending to faint. This is a stress reaction which will respond to opium in large doses [33]. In patients with chest wounds, profuse suppuration can develop, and opium is of great value in suppressing coughing and permitting the patient to sleep [34]. Opium was the only effective treatment for the pain following the agonizing procedure of grasping and pulling on a nasal polyp. There were also some remarks about the use of opium in the context of lithotomy. Bell is at pains to describe some of the variations in the clinical and pathological situation with bladder stones. In particular, he was concerned with the long-term adult sufferer, whose bladder had contracted and whose bladder wall had thickened. This individual would have suffered much pain and might have journeyed far to seek treatment. Such a patient should rest, sleep, and eat. Opiates were part of the treatment aimed at helping him recover his strength prior to surgery [35]. Then, as soon as the operation was complete, the patient was transported to a bed, where he was given opiates with a glass of wine and water [36]. Finally, Bell outlined a case of popliteal aneurysm, which progressed because the patient did not take it seriously. The clinical picture differed from that in modern textbooks. Bailey and Love describe a progressive pulsatile swelling behind the knee, which is largely asymptomatic, though it may be complicated by distal ischaemic symptoms due to thrombosis or distal emboli [37]. In Bell's case, the aneurysm increased in size rapidly and became increasingly painful and inflamed. It progressed until the patient asked for opiates to enable him to die quietly [38].

PHLEBOTOMY

There is no description of the technique of phlebotomy.

CONCLUSIONS

John Bell was a talented surgeon, and as is evident from his books, clearly a gifted teacher. His prose is clear, and his drawings illuminating. It must be a relief to know that the challenges he faced are unlikely to stress contemporary surgeons, in a world where early diagnosis and pre-operative imaging provide such an improved basis for surgical planning. His books also include a statement on the necessity of accepting the pain of an operation.

> *and I shall, I doubt not, prove to your conviction, that it is far better to suffer the salutary pains of operation and caustic than the unavoidable tortures of a disease, which, as soon as it becomes painful, is incurable [30].*

This is far less self-important than the quotation of Benjamin Bell on a similar topic (see Chapter 9). On the other hand, while the textbooks were valuable, they contained far too many criticisms of colleagues, which may have been overstated. It is believed that his more famous younger brother Charles was persuaded to move from Edinburgh by another brother (George) because of the difficulties he would face in Edinburgh from colleagues who had been disturbed by John [39].

John repeatedly stated that surgery should be fast when safe to minimize the time of suffering, but it should be slow when in regions of danger. In this context, pain should not be used as a motive to increase speed in situations that would put life at risk. This is a simply expressed concept of technical excellence that could hardly be improved.

REFERENCES

1. Bell J. *Oxford Dictionary of National Biography*. Oxford: Oxford University Press; 2004. (1763–1820).
2. Walls EW. John Bell, 1763–1820. *Medical History*. 1964; 8(1): 63–9.
3. Brown M. Surgery, Identity and Embodied Emotion: John Bell, James Gregory and the Edinburgh 'Medical War'. *History (Lond)*. 2019; 104: 19–41.
4. Gregory J. *Additional Memorial to the Managers of the Royal Infirmary*. Edinburgh: Murray & Cochrane; 1803.
5. Bell J. Preliminary Discourse on the Education and Duties of the Surgeon. In *The Principles of Surgery. I*. London: Thomas Tegg; 1826, pp. 1–14.
6. Bell J. Discourse VIII: Of Emphysema. In *The Principles of Surgery. I*. London: Thomas Tegg; 1826, pp. 437–51.

7. Bell J. Discourse IV: On the Various Uses of Bandages. In *The Principles of Surgery. I.* London: Thomas Tegg; 1826, pp. 170–6.
8. Bell J. Discourse 1: On Fractures of the Limbs – Introduction, Containing a History of the Opinions and Practices of the Older Surgeons. In *The Principles of Surgery. II.* London: Thomas Tegg; 1826, pp. 1–4.
9. Bell J. Discourse II – Cases for Illustration. In *The Principles of Surgery. II.* London: Thomas Tegg; 1826, pp. 599–612.
10. Bell J. Discourse I: On Tumours. In *The Excellency and Importance of this Department of Surgery. The Principles of Surgery. III.* London: Thomas Tegg; 1826, pp. 1–20.
11. Bell J. Discourse V: Of the Second Stage of Polypus. In *The Principles of Surgery. III.* London: Thomas Tegg; 1826, pp. 164–210.
12. Bell J. The History of the Operation of Lithotomy, and Criticism of the Different Operations - Preface. In *The Principles of Surgery. IV.* London: Thomas Tegg; 1826, pp. 1–21.
13. de Vet AC. Caries Cranii: Tuberculosis of the flat Bones of the Vault of the Skull. *Journal of Neurosurgery*. 1949; 6(4): 259–78.
14. Maxwell JH. Osteomyelitis of the Skull. In: Bancroft FW, Pilcher C, editors. *Surgical Treatment of the Nervous System*. Philadelphia, PA: J.B. Lippincott; 1946, pp. 92–108.
15. Bailey HH, Love RJM. *Bailey and Love's Short Practice of Surgery*. 27th ed. Boca Raton, FL: Taylor and Francis; 2018.
16. Wiseman R. *Eight Chirurgical Treatises*. London: Walthoe, J.; 1734.
17. Johnson T. *The Workes of the Famous Chirurgion Ambroise Pare: Translated out of the Latine and Compared with the French*. London: Richard Cotes; 1649.
18. Turner D. *The Art of Surgery*. London: Rivington, C; 1736.
19. Heister L. *A General System of Surgery in Three Parts*. London: W Innys; 1743.
20. Le Dran H-F. *The Operations in Surgery*. London: J Hodges at the Looking Glass; 1749.
21. Bell B. *A System of Surgery*. 6th ed. Edinburgh: Bell & Bradfute; 1796.
22. Bell J. *The Principles of Surgery*. London: Thomas Tegg; 1826.
23. Bell J. Discourse VI – Operation of the trepan. In *The Principles of Surgery. II.* London: Thomas Tegg; 1826, pp. 357–67.
24. Bell J. Discourse III: Position of the Patient. In *The Principles of Surgery. IV.* London: Thomas Tegg; 1826, pp. 246–7.
25. Bell J. Discourse II - Wounds Where Adhesion is not Easily Obtained, and of the Accidents by Which Adhesion is Hindered. In *The Principles of Surgery. II.* London: Thomas Tegg; 1826, pp. 78–83.
26. Bell J. Discourse III - Abuse of Poulices and Fomentations. In *The Principles of Surgery. I.* London: Thomas Tegg; 1826, pp. 90–4.
27. Bell J. Discourse III - The Skull not Absolutely Dependent on the Dura Mater. In *The Principles of Surgery. II.* London: Thomas Tegg; 1826, pp. 452–4.
28. Bell J. Discourse VII: Of Salivary Tumors. In *The Principles of Surgery. III.* London: Thomas Tegg; 1826, pp. 305–26.
29. Bell J. Discourse III: Of Ulcers. In *The Principles of Surgery. I.* London: Thomas Tegg; 1826, pp. 115–21.
30. Bell J. Discourse IV: Of Tumors of the Nostrils, Gums, and Throat. In *The Principles of Surgery. III.* London: Thomas Tegg; 1826, pp. 117–51.
31. Bell J. Discourse VI: Of Tumors of the Gums, Lips, Cheeks and Throat. In *The Principles of Surgery. III.* London: Thomas Tegg; 1826, pp. 224–304.
32. Bell J. Discourse VII: Of the Aneurism by Anastomosis. In *The Principles of Surgery. III.* London: Thomas Tegg; 1826, pp. 326–48.

33. Bell J. Discourse III - Hospital Gangrene. In *The Principles of Surgery. I.* London: Thomas Tegg; 1826, pp. 136–53.
34. Bell J. Discourse VIII - Supporting the Patient Under Profuse Suppuration. In *The Principles of Surgery. I.* London: Thomas Tegg; 1826, pp. 453–5.
35. Bell J. Discourse III: Importance of Careful Examination Before Operating. In *The Principles of Surgery. IV.* London: Thomas Tegg; 1826, pp. 238–41.
36. Bell J. Discourse III: Of Bleeding After the Operation. In *The Principles of Surgery. IV.* London: Thomas Tegg; 1826, pp. 262–4.
37. Sayers R, Davies RSM. Popliteal Aneurysm. In *Bailey and Love's Short Practice of Surgery*. 27th ed. Boca Raton, FL: Taylor and Francis; 2018, pp. 965–6.
38. Bell J. Discourse III: Progress of a Politeal Aneurism. In *The Principles of Surgery. IV.* London: Thomas Tegg; 1826, pp. 363–5.
39. Gordon-Taylor G. The life and times of Sir Charles Bell. *The Annals of The Royal College of Surgeons of England.* 1956; 18(1): 1–24.

11 Surgical Pain – Transition to the Nineteenth Century: Astley Paston Cooper (1768–1841)

INTRODUCTION

Biographical information about the distinguished surgeons previously mentioned in this book is mostly absent or at least limited. Astley Paston Cooper, by contrast, has been the subject of quite a few biographies of varying length, dating back to just after his death [1–6]. This is a measure of the impact he had on the history and development of surgery. He was the fourth son and sixth child of a well-to-do British parson located in Brook Hall, a few miles from Norwich, which at the time was the second city of the country, (today it is No. 128). He had a comfortable and loving childhood. He was not an eager schoolboy with his nose to books. On the contrary, he was a lively young ne'er-do-well, much admired by friends and family [3, 4]. He had an uncle who was a surgeon in London, which was part of the reason for him to study in the capital, but he did not study with his family. Instead, he lodged with an excellent surgeon, Henry Cline, who, after a while, engaged Cooper's interest so that thereafter he became hard-working and inquisitive. In addition, Cline was a student of the great pioneer of science applied to surgery, John Hunter. Cooper also came to be influenced by Hunter and spent a lifetime dissecting and improving his knowledge of anatomy, an intimate knowledge of which is the essential basis for operating. In addition, he adopted Hunter's notion that knowledge was not based on the teachings of the past but on direct experience and observation. This was a vital basis for learning how to be a better surgeon.

So why has Cooper remained such a subject of continuing interest? During his lifetime, he was famous for the quality of his lectures on anatomy. He was part of the group of surgeons associated with John Hunter, who introduced a method of increasing knowledge of surgery and anatomy. It was said of him:

As a teacher Sir Astley Cooper has never been excelled by any English surgeon [7].

He also made a number of important contributions to the practice of surgery. He was a pioneer of proximal artery ligation in the treatment of aneurysms. He was the first to describe the transversalis fascia, which is important in hernia surgery. He also described an eponymous ligament attached to the superior aspect of the pubic bone. Cooper's ligament in the breast provides support for the fat and glandular tissue and contributes to the shape and consistency of the breasts.

DOI: 10.1201/9781003748816-11

Cooper gradually acquired a huge practice and was very successful, not only clinically and academically but also financially. In the prime of his career, his income was not less than £15,000 and his manservant 'Charles' was said to make £600 by getting potential patients appointments out of turn [8]. In his final years, it is said that Cooper's annual income reached £21,000 [5]. That is more than £2,000,000 in today's money [9]. It might reasonably be expected that such success would result in jealousy and criticism, particularly at a time when the medical press was a good deal less guarded than it is today. However, with the exception of one modern, rather spiteful paper [4], his contemporaries were consistent in their praise [8]. As has been mentioned before in this book, the relationship between surgeon and patient is within the context of the surgical management, inevitably uneven. The patient needs help; the surgeon can hopefully provide it. This is a situation that easily leads to paternalism and arrogance. While confidence is an absolute requirement for a surgeon, it remains a lifelong battle to avoid tipping over from confidence to arrogance. Thus, it is yet another measure of the quality of the man that his courtesy to patients was repeatedly remarked upon. His kindness was evidenced by his seeing poor patients in the early morning at his home without charging a fee [10]. In addition, he arranged for five of his assistants to travel to Belgium to help in the treatment of wounded soldiers after the Battle of Waterloo. He was the only London surgeon to do so. He also treated wounded officers for free in the subsequent years [11]. Thus, while he had a huge income, he could hardly be accused of greed or meanness. Indeed, his personality was his greatest strength, gaining him the trust of the range of social classes from King George IV to the lowest in the land.

THE IMPACT OF FEAR ON SURGICAL RESULTS

In his opening lecture, Cooper acknowledges the importance of fear in a number of anecdotes.

> *But fear has the greatest influence in destroying your best efforts to cure injuries or diseases... Not long since, a person came to me from the country...When I informed him he had the stone, he said, "I hope not, for I can never submit to an operation." ... he died in a few days after.*

When he was a student with Mr. Cline, he recollected the following patient.

> *A lady consulted for a tumour in her breast, which he recommended to be removed. She said, she was sure that the operation would kill her; but it was observed, that the removal of such a tumour was generally attended with little danger. Although unwilling to submit and strongly impressed with the idea that the operation would be fatal in its issue, her friends prevailed upon her to consent: and, when I mention Mr. Cline as the operator, it is unnecessary to say, that it was done with all that skill and caution could effect. She died on the same day, only an hour after the operation; and it was found, that she had arranged her family and domestic concerns in such a manner, that no confusion should arise from what she thought her inevitable doom [12].*

Later on in the book he mentions the consequences of timidity on the treatment of perianal fistulae.

> *Of the Cure by Seton.—Timid persons prefer this mode of treatment to the knife, although in the one case the irritation is long continued, and in the other the pain is only of a few minutes' continuance. That it succeeds, in some instances, I have known; for some of my patient's, having submitted to this remedy, returned to me well. My objection to it is, that the irritation it produces is liable to occasion other abscesses, whilst healing that for which it is employed [13].*

At a later date, Cooper recalled the misfortune of a private soldier who was celebrating a new monarch.

> *Mr. T. aet. 31, a private in the Newbury Volunteer Cavalry, had been dining at Newbury with the troop, to celebrate the coronation of his present Majesty. When returning home at a late hour with some others of the troop, they were attacked by a number of the Queen's partizans, and during the affray which succeeded, Mr. T. received a violent blow from a brickbat on the superior part of the frontal bone, which caused a depression of a portion of the bone, and considerable haemorrhage. Mr. Hemsted, surgeon, at Newbury, was sent for to attend him, and directed that he should be freely bled and purged; which relieved him so much, that at the end of four days he returned home apparently well. Mr. Hemsted, however, told him he would be very fortunate if he felt no further inconvenience from the accident, and advised him to keep particularly quiet and sober*
>
> *On the 20th of January 1822, exactly six months from the receipt of the injury, he had an epileptic fit; Mr. H. was called to visit him, and recommended the same plan of treatment. The fits, however, returned once or twice every fortnight; and oftener, if he exerted himself, or was guilty of any excess. Mr. H. told him, that he could not be cured without having the depressed portion of bone removed; to which he was averse, and came to town to consult me, when I confirmed the opinion of Mr. H. The patient still refused to undergo any operation at that period. The fits increased in frequency; and on the 30th of July 1822, having had two, he became much alarmed, and sent for Mr. Hemsted to remove the portion of depressed bone, which Mr. H. did with a trephine. He speedily recovered from the operation, and has not since had any return of the epileptic fits [14].*

THE PAIN OF SURGERY

Cooper, in a statement early in the book, pointed out that inflammation made tissues more pain sensitive, so that the degree of pain experienced during an operation is related to the degree of inflammation [15]. This was an original and valuable insight. Cooper, as will be demonstrated, adapted his technique to minimize pain. However, he also noted a number of situations in which reducing the intensity of pain was simply impossible.

A paronychia is a soft tissue infection around a fingernail. If it progresses to pus formation, this needs to be drained. Today this is done under local anaesthesia and may involve removal of some of the nail adjacent to the infection. It is a very painful condition. Cooper wrote:

It sometimes happens, however, that the sore is so exceedingly irritable… in such cases, what I do is this: with a pair of scissors I slit up the nail on the side where the disease exists, and then, with forceps, turn back, and sometimes completely remove, the divided portion. This is a very painful operation certainly, but I have known persons get well by this treatment in ten days, when the complaint had for months resisted every other [16].

A urogenital condition where the pain of treatment is unavoidable was amputation of the penis for a carcinoma at the distal end of the organ. The excision was unavoidably agonizing, but on the other hand, it was done very quickly, and the pain was soon over [17]. Following amputation, the residual distal end should not be covered with skin as this could lead to retention of urine. While the end was granulating, a bougie was kept in the urethra to prevent stricture [17].

Cooper's descriptions of operations reveal an obsessive determination to do everything as perfectly as possible. No other author had described the immobilization for lithotomy in greater detail, concluding the description with the remark:

These bandages prevent the patient from making any movements likely to impede the operation, or occasion danger during its performance [18].

He insisted that patients' general health should be checked prior to accepting them for lithotomy. This would reduce the mortality of the procedure. The use of the forceps during lithotomy should be as gentle as possible, not only to minimize pain but also to avoid injury to the sensitive bladder epithelium [18].

Cooper outlined a number of technical details aimed at minimizing the distress occasioned by an operation. He was concerned with not just the pain but also the consequences of an ugly scar in the neck following drainage of an abscess. He mentioned that this was a particular difficulty for young women, since an ugly scar could have a negative effect on their chances of marriage. To this end, he used a small blade, making a skin opening as tiny as possible, with two advantages. It was less frightening to the patient, and the scar was much less visible [19]. This was an innovation.

Patients with a hydrocele might not be suitable for a formal operation because of either poor general health or fear of the procedure. Cooper bowed to the circumstances or the patient's wishes and treated them with tapping [20].

If during castration, the testis was attached to the skin, he chose to remove the attached skin with the testis, thereby avoiding an unnecessary and painful dissection to separate the two tissues [21].

With tuberculous nodules, he recommended excision. If left untouched, these lesions could ulcerate, which was a most distressing and painful condition worth avoiding even if the operation could not preserve or prolong life [22].

In the treatment of perianal fistula, he described a detailed and precise post-operative management. Lint should be introduced into the wound *at once* and compressed until all bleeding stops. This was followed by a sequence of poultice, probing, and after a few days the lint would separate. Gradually, the granulation tissue filled the cavity. Introducing the lint on the second day or later would lead to pain, infection, and suppuration.

Then he had advice on how to simplify haemorrhoidectomy. Early in his career, he favoured excision of haemorrhoids, but with increasing experience, he came to prefer a ligature, and he had detailed advice on how the ligature should be applied [13].

He also proffered advice on how to reduce pain during surgical procedures to the mouth and nose. He operated nasal polyps by introducing closed scissors into the nostril to identify the attachment of the polyp. The scissors were then open, and the polyp attachment was cut through. He specifically mentioned that the approach had critics who disliked it because of excessive bleeding. He remarked that could only occur if the operation were performed in an 'indiscreet' manner. He rejected the use of a ligature because of technical difficulty and the uncertainty of including the entire polyp.

Finally, Cooper provided helpful advice on the performance of tonsillectomy, an operation undertaken not because of the presence of an enlarged tonsil but rather because of persistent conservative treatment resistant symptoms. If a tonsil was peduncular, then a ligature might be tightened around its root. This was left in situ until it ulcerated through the tonsil after about a week. Cooper also discussed multiple ligatures passed with needles through the base of the tonsil if that was broad. However, he found that technique inefficient. He preferred excision using scissors and suggested this should be undertaken bit by bit, and not completed in a single session [23].

THE PAIN OF CAUTERY

Cautery receives two mentions. It is suggested in passing that it may have a part to play in some lip cancers [24] and in the management of poisoned bites, as from a rabid animal [25]. There is absolutely no other consideration of the method.

ANALGESICS

The prescription of opium refers to use of the drug taken by mouth. Cooper would have seen many patients with long-lasting inflammation, and he provided thoughts on the underlying mechanisms which included the interaction of mind and body, and more physical changes explained in terms of humoural physiology. Opium was the preferred medicine for this condition. In abscesses, opium was favoured for reducing irritation and was also considered to expedite suppuration. It also provided the best symptom relief for the very painful irritable ulcer, which was an ulcer with uneven granulations and a discharge of a mixture of blood and pus. A grain of opium morning and evening provided the most effective pain relief [19]. Cooper describes gangrenous ulcers with livid margins, containing small vesicles and blisters and the surface of which was free of discharge. They required intensive local care to separate the dead tissue. Fifty drops of nitric acid in two pints of distilled water was favoured for this purpose. Twenty drops of tincture of opium were given three times a day to alleviate the associated pain and distress [16]. If gangrene developed, the dose could be elevated to twenty drops every four hours [26]. If suppuration developed in an injured joint, opium would be needed [27].

Opium was also administered for indications not related to inflammation. It was useful in managing the systemic reaction to surgery following an operation for popliteal aneurysm [28]. A patient who had endured a hydatid cyst in the breast for two years accepted surgery when the lump entered a phase of rapid growth. Prior to surgery, opium was used for the pain. Tuberculous nodules could become large, and they were extremely painful so that opium was part of the pre-operative management prior to the operation, which was the only treatment that could provide relief. Cooper also described what he called an irritable tumour of the breast. This occurred in young women and varied in size with the menstrual cycle. It did not require surgery but was painful enough to need opium [29]. After an operation for an inguinal hernia, violent diarrhoea could occur, and opium was useful in its suppression [30]. Opium was also given when pressure on a strangulated hernia failed to reduce it [31]. If internal haemorrhoids arose as a complication of diarrhoea, opium could be useful [13]. Opium was also used as a palliative in the sad situation of an untreatable malignant nasal polyp [23].

There were a number of urogenital conditions in which opium was of use. It was recommended for ureteric colic [32]. It was useful for the discomfort and systemic disturbance following lithotomy in children. Apparently, opium had a specific application for urethral calculi. A catheter was introduced as far as the membranous urethra. When this met a calculus embedded at that location, the catheter was withdrawn to be replaced by a bougie. The patient was given opium together with antimony tartrate for thirty to sixty minutes. During this period, the patient should sit in water as hot as he could tolerate. Then removal of the bougie would often be followed by the stone [33].

Finally, opium had a place in the management of trauma. It facilitated reduction of a dislocated hip [33] and was useful in the management of ankle dislocations [34]. It was useful in countering the general debility following wounds [25], contused wounds and puncture wounds [35]. In laryngeal injuries, patients received enemas which included opium. If the subsequent evacuation were excessive, opium would help reduce the excess [36]. In addition, if when lying in bed waiting for a tendon to heal, a patient becomes restless or suffered pain, opium could come to his/her aid [27]. Finally, opium was given for severe headache persisting for months after a cranial injury [37].

PHLEBOTOMY

Cooper found an indication for phlebotomy in particular in the management of inflammations. However, he was perhaps one of the earliest to recommend that the procedure was not always beneficial and should be used with circumspection. Scepsis about phlebotomy had been growing. Benjamin Bell's teacher James Hill had been close to a Dumfries physician called Ebenezer Gilchrist (1708 to 1774), who doubted that bloodletting did much good [38]. Change was clearly in the air.

CONCLUSION

The clarity of Cooper's text is noteworthy. All his expressions indicate care and thoroughness of a man who did what he could to minimize pain and comply with patients' wishes. He clearly had great social and professional gifts. What is surprising is his assessment of himself. The remarks are taken from his notebooks. They are in the third person, and it has been suggested that it is because they were intended for a biographer. Nonetheless, they are his own opinions on himself.

> *Sir Astley Cooper was a good anatomist, but never was a good operator where delicacy was required. He felt too much before he began ever to make a perfect operator. "For the operation of cataract he was quite unfitted by nature [1].*

It would seem therefore that he was a most admirable human being in both his private and professional life [5]. He approved of adequate doses of opium for pain with the dose guided by its efficacy. He showed an open attitude at least in one instance where he changed his opinion on how to treat haemorrhoids with increasing experience. He managed the poor without charging a fee. He also demonstrated his consideration in another way. Surgeons vary in their consideration of post-operative scars. Cooper showed consideration with abscesses in the neck using a small knife blade to minimize scarring, which in young women could damage the chances of getting married.

Finally, in a variety of situations, he operated with a technique that, while not pain free, minimized pain as far as possible.

REFERENCES

1. Cooper BB. *The Life of Sir Astley Cooper, Bart.* Kibdib: John W. Parker; 1843.
2. Unknown. Brief Memoir of Sir Astley Paston Cooper, Bart. *Lancet*. 1849; 1(1): 1–3.
3. Cooper AP. *Oxford Dictionary of National Biography*. Oxford: Oxford University Press; 2008, p. 1–7.
4. Burch D. Astley Paston Cooper (1768–1841): Anatomist, Radical and Surgeon. *Journal of the Royal Society of Medicine*. 2010; 103: 505–8.
5. Burch D. *Digging up the Dead*. London: Chatto & Windus; 2007.
6. Brock RC. *The Life and Work of Astley Cooper*. London: E. & S. Livingstone; 1952.
7. Brock RC. His Daily Work. In *The Life and Work of Astley Cooper*. London: E. & S. Livingstone; 1952, pp. 28–31.
8. Guthrie D. XVIII Century Medicine (Continued). In *A History of Medicine*. London: Thomas Nelson and Sons Ltd; 1960, pp. 235–65.
9. Anon. Bank of England Inflation Calculator. 2025. Available from: https://www.bankofengland.co.uk/monetary-policy/inflation/inflation-calculator
10. Cooper BB. Chapter XIII. In *The Life of Sir Astley Cooper, Bart. 1*. Kibdib: John W. Parker; 1843, pp. 226–46.
11. Cooper BB. Chapter VII. In *The Life of Sir Astley Cooper, Bart. 2*. Kibdib: John W. Parker; 1843, pp. 180–207.
12. Cooper A. On Irritation. In *The Principles and Practice of Surgery*. London: E. Portwine; 1835, pp. 9–23.
13. Cooper A. Of Fistula in Ano. In *The Principles and Practice of Surgery*. London: E. Portwine; 1835, pp. 293–302.
14. Cooper A. Compression of the Brain. In *The Principles and Practice of Surgery*. London: E. Portwine; 1835, pp. 125–38.
15. Cooper A. On Inflammation. In *The Principles and Practice of Surgery*. London: E. Portwine; 1835, pp. 23–33.
16. Cooper A. On Ulcers. In *The Principles and Practice of Surgery*. London: E. Portwine; 1835, pp. 84–96.

17. Cooper A. Cancer Labii. In *The Principles and Practice of Surgery*. London: E. Portwine; 1835, pp. 326–8.
18. Cooper A. On the Operation of Lithotomy. In *The Principles and Practice of Surgery*. London: E. Portwine; 1835, pp. 258–80.
19. Cooper A. On Ulceration. In *The Principles and Practice of Surgery*. London: E. Portwine; 1835, pp. 61–74.
20. Cooper A. Of the Operations for the Cure of the Hydrocele. In *The Principles and Practice of Surgery*. London: E. Portwine; 1835, pp. 198–205.
21. Cooper A. On the Simple Chronic Enlargement of the Testis. In *The Principles and Practice of Surgery*. London: E. Portwine; 1835, pp. 215–24.
22. Cooper A. On the Treatment of the Scirrhous Tubercle. In *The Principles and Practice of Surgery*. London: E. Portwine; 1835, pp. 236–48.
23. Cooper A. Of Polypus of the Nose. In *The Principles and Practice of Surgery*. London: E. Portwine; 1835, pp. 302–10.
24. Cooper A. Of Harelip. In *The Principles and Practice of Surgery*. London: E. Portwine; 1835, pp. 321–31.
25. Cooper A. On Wounds. In *The Principles and Practice of Surgery*. London: E. Portwine; 1835, pp. 409–14.
26. Cooper A. On Gangrene. In *The Principles and Practice of Surgery*. London: E.Portwine; 1835, pp. 96–112.
27. Cooper A. On Wounds of Joints. In *The Principles and Practice of Surgery*. London: E. Portwine; 1835, pp. 454–62.
28. Cooper A. On Aneurism. In *The Principles and Practice of Surgery*. London: E. Portwine; 1835, pp. 165–75.
29. Cooper A. On Diseases of the Breast. In *The Principles and Practice of Surgery*. London: E. Portwine; 1835, pp. 224–36.
30. Cooper A. Operation for Inguinal Hernia. In *The Principles and Practice of Surgery*. London: E. Portwine; 1835, pp. 366–81.
31. Cooper A. On Femoral Herniæ. In *The Principles and Practice of Surgery*. London: E. Portwine; 1835, pp. 381–91.
32. Cooper A. Of Urinary Calculi. In *The Principles and Practice of Surgery*. London: E. Portwine; 1835, pp. 248–58.
33. Cooper A. On Disclocations of the Hip. In *The Principles and Practice of Surgery*. London: E. Portwine; 1835, pp. 503–31.
34. Cooper A. On Disclocations of the Ankle. In *The Principles and Practice of Surgery*. London: E. Portwine; 1835, pp. 549–74.
35. Cooper A. On Contused Wounds. In *The Principles and Practice of Surgery*. London: E. Portwine; 1835, pp. 415–24.
36. Cooper A. On Wounds of Veins. In *The Principles and Practice of Surgery*. London: E. Portwine; 1835, pp. 435–53.
37. Cooper A. On Wounds of the Brain. In *The Principles and Practice of Surgery*. London: E. Portwine; 1835, pp. 139–55.
38. Gilchrist E. *Oxford Dictionary of National Biography*. Oxford: Oxford University Press; 2004.

12 Surgical Pain – Transition to the Nineteenth Century: Robert Liston (1794–1847)

INTRODUCTION

The character of Robert Liston was in marked contrast to that of Astley Cooper. He was serious, not particularly sociable, and did not magnetize people with his charisma. He was born in Ecclesmachan, about twelve miles west of the centre of Edinburgh. He appears to have come from a gifted family. His younger brother David became Professor of Oriental languages at Edinburgh. While his father Henry was the minister of the parish, he was also something of an expert in the design of pipe organs [1]. Robert entered the University of Edinburgh at the age of fourteen in 1808, where he studied Latin and won a prize. At the age of sixteen, in 1810, he started his medical education as assistant to Dr John Barclay, an anatomist. In 1814, he became a House Surgeon (Intern) at the Edinburgh Royal Infirmary. In 1816, he went to study in London, returned home in 1818, and in the same year was admitted as a Fellow of the Royal College of Surgeons of Edinburgh [1, 2]. From then to 1828, Liston gained a reputation as an anatomist and surgeon, and quarrelled constantly with the authorities. When he was not appointed to the chair of surgery in Edinburgh, he departed for London in 1834 to take up the chair of surgery at the newly founded institution, which in time would become known as the University College Hospital. In 1835, he was appointed Professor of Clinical Surgery. In 1837, he published his 'Practical Surgery', which teaches us so much of his principles [1, 2].

The introduction to 'Practical Surgery' states a number of notions and axioms with unsurpassed lucidity and unmatched passion. He was famed for the elegance and speed of his operating, much like a concert pianist is celebrated for the effortlessness of a dazzling performance. Yet in both instances, the public performance would be based on a lifetime of preparation. What is so impressive about Liston is the clarity with which he states the requirements of preparation and their application in practice.

He quotes the French surgeon Desault's remark '*the simplicity of an operation is the measure of its perfection.*' This remark is followed by a specification of the simplicity of instruments and dressings that would prove optimal. He insists that the indications to operate had become stricter than in the past, reducing the need to operate in many cases. He then states with passion his view on the undertaking an operation.

> *It behoves, therefore– indeed it is the bounden duty of every one engaging in the practice of our profession, in addition to a correct knowledge of the science of surgery, –*

DOI: 10.1201/9781003748816-12

> *the causes, symptoms, and consequences of disease, the signs of injuries, the morbid changes in the tissues involved,– to make, moreover, the art of operating the subject of most careful and diligent study [3].*

He has more to say on the principles of performing an operation:

> *The art of operating has, even by many of those in prominent situations, been too lightly considered, and too little practised on the dead body. The foundation of the study of the art of operating must be laid in the dissecting-room, and it is only when we have acquired dexterity on the dead subject, that we can be justified in interfering with the living. Many poor creatures have been sacrificed in consequence of the ignorance, carelessness, and self-sufficiency even of scientific professors, who have either despised or neglected the study of surgical anatomy, the consideration of the casualties which may arise during the various operations, and the due education of their fingers. The infliction of unnecessary pain, through want of adroitness in the use of instruments, and consequent protraction of the operative procedure — the hazarding in the slightest degree the safety of any one who puts confidence in us, and entrusts to us his life, or of one who, as in public practice, is, by chance, and without the means of appeal, thrown upon our care — cannot by any means be palliated or defended — and is, in point of fact, highly criminal [3].*

He tells us that successful surgery requires familiarity with anatomy and comfortable dexterity with the instruments. This is learned in the dissecting room. He emphasized the need to keep the pain of surgery to a minimum. This is in part achieved by reducing the time of an operation, which requires dexterity [3]. Having laid out the responsibilities of the surgeon during surgery, he then moves to the interaction with the patient. He states:

> *the first consideration that ought to occupy attention, is the state of mind and feelings of the sufferer, and the condition of the digestive organs and circulating system [4].*

If all is in order, then:

> *his stomach, bowels, and kidneys being all in good order, and his circulation quiet, — the less delay in resorting to operative procedure, and the shorter the period of uncertainty and suspense in which the patient is kept, the better [4].*

In the first five pages of his book, he lays out the technical and humanitarian principles of surgery in a manner upon which it would be difficult to improve. However, unlike the surgeons in the previous four chapters, Liston does not write about the techniques required to convince patients that an operation was necessary. He begins his account with a patient who is prepared for the knife. There is one other detail of Liston's book which bears mention. There are many well-drawn illustrations to illuminate the text. They are perhaps not of the same elegance as those of John Bell, but they contrast well with the works of Latta, Benjamin Bell, and Astley Cooper, which include no comparable images.

PAIN OF SURGERY

Liston's technical adaptations for the reduction of pain are both general, applying to any situation, and specific, applying to exclusive pathological processes and locations. The general techniques are considered first. He considered details of the skin incisions, being only the second surgeon to do so. Astley Cooper had insisted that incisions in the necks of women should be kept as small as possible, to reduce the cosmetic damage. However, he did not set out a statement of principles. Liston provided two relevant comments, the first related to the nature of tissue sensibility:

> *All incisions, more especially through the skin, the most sensitive part of the animal machine, should be effected with rapidity, and in such a way as to give as little pain and shock to the nervous system as possible [4].*

This was followed by a statement on the method to be employed:

> *The cutaneous tissues, and in many instances the subjacent parts, should be divided by a single incision, rather than that the patient should be tormented, and the feelings of those who witness the proceeding hurt, by the process being effected bit by bit, as it were, by slow and tedious procedure [4].*

He went a step further by recommending the correct way to hold the knife with firm fingers and a flexible wrist. In addition, he specified the angle of the knife to skin. He illustrated his intention with a reference to the skill of a soldier with the comment:

> *And if agility and address are to be acquired by constant study and practice in the elegant exercise of the small sword, why should not "grace and splendour," as was the boast of Hildanus, be equally attainable by the surgeon, and by similar means? [4].*

All of these statements underline the humanity that informs Liston's entire approach to his work. There are a number of other general pieces of advice concerning surgical technique. No matter how deep abscesses were, they should be drained early. This reduced the duration of pain suffered. Drainage must be free, and an opening of an inch was no more painful than a smaller perforation. Multiple incisions may be needed. Abscesses should not be squeezed, since that involves unnecessary pain. It may also be remembered that if an incision must be extended, it may be preferable to incise from within outwards.

There was a belief at his time that when a blood vessel was closed with a ligature, it would resorb of itself. Liston believed ligatures could be troublesome, causing inflammation and suppuration. Thus, in situations where swift wound healing was expected, one end of the ligature should remain accessible, so that it may be used in the removal of the retained material. In wounds where skin adaptation was not possible and closure might be delayed, both ends of a ligature might be cut. He also insisted on the same point as my teacher Richard Johnson, a British neurosurgeon celebrated for the quality of his surgical technique. Always prefer to use a knife in the division of living tissue, and avoid scissors, which compress as they cut and which would be more painful for the patient [4]. In addition, he noted that properly handled knives could be used close to blood vessels [5]. This is further evidence to permit the knife in preference to scissors when dissecting. Moreover, a sharp knife may be used to shave exuberant granulations. This was less painful than the use of caustics. Another way to reduce suffering was to avoid caustics that were too powerful, such as antimony chloride or potassium carbonate. Liston preferred zinc chloride, which should be applied while at the same time giving the patient oral opium preparations to counteract the pain [6]. Finally, Liston makes the point in keeping with Ambroise Parė [7] that:

No harm can accrue from small foreign bodies remaining, and the chance is that sooner or later they will become apparent, so as to be certainly and easily removed [8].

Then there were quite a few specific technical adaptations, starting with the head and its contents. He rejected the use of ligatures for tonsillectomy because it was difficult, tedious, painful, and unnecessary. Radical tonsillectomy was not needed. A partial removal of the tonsil could be achieved with a sharp knife, gently resecting tissue up to the level of the soft palate. Bleeding was not a problem. This procedure was not as painful as extracting a tooth. He reduced the pain of parotid surgery by carrying the dissection deep to the lower boundary of the disease, thereby finding supplying blood vessels that could be controlled, thereby avoiding repeated needs to stop and arrest bleeding during the dissection [6]. There was also advice for those dealing with the lachrymal apparatus. One of the causes of excessive tear production is blockage of the nasolacrimal duct. Relieving this block involved the introduction of a probe of the correct shape. Dexterity in achieving this involved two aspects. These were the use of a small, specially constructed steel sound and practice on dead bodies in the laboratory. This is yet a repetition of the previously stated principles that were the basis for Liston's success [9]. One other detail he mentioned is reminiscent of my own experience. Emergency tracheotomies are often performed by junior resident staff, who frequently complained that the procedure was difficult because of the bleeding. Indeed, the anterior cervical veins in this situation are often dramatically dilated due to increased intrathoracic pressure. But, when the young colleagues were asked why they had touched the veins, they seemed to think it was unavoidable. This is not the case, and, as Liston advises, the surgeon should avoid the division of any superficial vein [9].

It is important to note that Liston was not obsessed with speed. John Bell, in the Short Preliminary Discourse to his text on surgery, harking back to medieval times:

I would say rather: with Guy de Chauliac,-'Sit audax in· securis, timidus in periculis; let him cut rapidly, and dexterously where all is safe, slowly and cautiously where there is danger[10].

Liston followed this principle to the letter as shown in this following statement about mastectomy.

This is a disease in which no half measures will answer; and if, after a severe struggle, a patient has made up her mind to submit to the pain and risk of a very dreadful operation, in the expectation of saving herself from after suffering, and enjoying an immunity from a terrible disease, it is not fair, by slovenliness or carelessness, to throw away a chance, or in any way to endanger recurrence of the mischief. The operation is one which must be conducted deliberately and conscientiously; as, indeed, ought to be the case in undertaking operations of any kind, and in any situation. The duration of the proceeding must not be considered. Many operations can be done well, and quickly too, and fully as well when quickly. But this is not one of these; the extirpation should be performed with a thorough determination to free the patient from the whole of the diseased structure [6].

There was further advice for the surgeon operating on the genitourinary system and in the perineum. He reflects on vascular tumours of the lower bowel with the remark:

Something has been said lately by one or more of the Dublin surgeons about vascular tumours of the lower bowel, and the necessity of applying very strong nitric acid to destroy them. I have not met with any disease in these parts requiring so severe, painful, and dangerous a proceeding [9].

Liston recommended trusses for the treatment of varicocele. He points out that while the treatment will not lead to a radical cure it can relieve most of the discomfort in most cases and avoids a very painful operation. Liston wrote a thesis on urethral stricture for his Fellowship of the Royal College of Surgeons of Edinburgh. In his 'Practical Surgery' he wrote:

The operation of introducing a catheter, through what has been called an impermeable stricture, is without doubt the most difficult in the whole range of surgical operations, and demands all the prudence, science, and skill of a master. The art can only be acquired, and that gradually, by frequent practice.

He suggested that strictures are often the consequence of urethral injury following awkward attempts to catheterize patients with retention of urine. He was also involved in developing the instrumentation used to perform lithotrity, whereby bladder stones could be crushed in the bladder and either passed with the urine or washed out. This was clearly far less painful than a lithotomy, which involved a perineal incision and an incision in the bladder. Liston retained lithotomy as the treatment for children, or for adults who had ignored their stone, enabling it to become very large. He further insisted that immobilization for lithotomy was of vital importance and provided the most detailed instructions as to how this could be achieved. Finally, he maintained that lithotomy should only be undertaken by surgeons with great experience in the procedure [11].

There is one other practical detail concerning operating on children. A child to be operated for hare lip was to be placed on a nurse's knee after being wrapped and pinned up in a large cloth, so that hands and feet were perfectly confined and all struggling prevented.

PAIN OF CAUTERY

Liston's opening remark on cautery is:

> *In the modern and more approved practice of surgery, cauteries are seldom, if ever, had recourse to for arresting haemorrhage. The proceeding is appalling, cruel, and after all not much to be trusted to. Neither, happily, is the hot iron, nor actual fire in any form, much, if at all, used as a means of cure, in this country, at least by surgical practitioners [4].*

He also specified that caustic substances need to be used only with adequate expertise. Their effects were not interchangeable but specific and when applied should be chosen with that specificity in mind [4]. There are a few references in the text to the use of actual or potential cautery, but the use of cautery was clearly not a significant part of Liston's practice.

ANALGESICS

Opium was used to treat the pain of some diseases but was not given to reduce the pain of an operation [6].

PHLEBOTOMY

Liston gives a precise description of his technique of venesection and the management of complications. He insisted that damage to an artery is rare, but if it occurs, as a 'consequence of careless venesection' ligation is the treatment. His views on injuries to tendons and nerves are unlike those of any predecessor. He wrote:

> *The wounds of tendons do not deserve notice, nor even those of nerves; the former can scarcely be injured in the operation, and if they were, would not, in all probability, lead to any bad consequence. Partial division of branches of the cutaneous nerves has given rise to painful feelings in the limb, and to general disturbance of the nervous system. But such occurrences are rare; they may be treated by general means, or, if need be, the original wound may be slightly enlarged. No regular dissection at the bend of the arm, as has been proposed, can ever be warranted. Benjamin Bell would have had us almost sever the extremity by incisions through fascia, muscles, and tendons, even to the periosteum, in search of nerves supposed to have been injured in venesection [5].*

Liston's experience is at odds with that of every reporting surgeon from Celsus onwards. He gives no explanation for this difference, and it is impossible to know with any certainty why it was so. It is, however, possible to speculate, and it seems not improbable that in the rare event that an injury to a tendon or nerve occurred, the elegance and precision of his technique meant that the total extent of the injury was much less than that of other surgeons, who experienced the induction of considerable pain.

CONCLUSION

Liston's text expresses a close-to-ideal understanding of the purpose of surgery, and with unusual clarity, he expresses the means with which this may be carried out. Relieving pain is central to his concepts. The methods used to achieve this required long-term study and practice, in the same way as professional musicians and athletes practice before performing. This practice provided dexterity, which could reduce the time of an operation and thus the duration of suffering. Accurate knowledge of the anatomy of the parts to be operated permitted confidence and reduced hesitation. Even for those without Liston's legendary dexterity, any surgeon can confirm that speed is achieved by doing only what is intended. In other words, if you want to stop a vessel bleeding, you do it at the first attempt and avoid injuring other vessels, the closure of which delays the procedure.

REFERENCES

1. England RCoSo. *Details for Liston, Robert (1794–1847)*. 2007. Available from: https://livesonline.rcseng.ac.uk/client/en_GB/lives/search/results?qu=Liston%2C+Robert&te=ASSET
2. Liston R. *Oxford Dictionary of National Biography*. Oxford: Oxford University Press; 2004.
3. Liston R. Introduction. In *Practical Surgery*. London: John Churchill; 1846, pp. 1–4.
4. Liston R. Division by the Knife, Ligature, and Escharotics. In *Practical Surgery*. London: John Churchill; 1846, pp. 5–29.
5. Liston R. Injuries and Diseases of Blood Vessels. In *Practical Surgery*. London: John Churchill; 1846, pp. 175–233.
6. Liston R. Morbid Growths and Enlargements. In *Practical Surgery*. London: John Churchill; 1846, pp. 269–352.
7. Johnson T. Of Wounds in Generall. In *The Workes of the Famous Chirurgion Ambroise Pare: Translated out of the Latine and Compared with the French*. London: Richard Cotes; 1649, pp. 252–5.
8. Liston R. Injuries and Diseases of Integument and Cellular Tissue. In *Practical Surgery*. London: John Churchill; 1846, pp. 234–49.
9. Liston R. Injuries and Diseases of Mucous Canals and Cavities. In *Practical Surgery*. London: John Churchill; 1846, pp. 393–443.
10. Bell J. Preliminary Discourse on the Education and Duties of the Surgeon. In *The Principles of Surgery. I*. London: Thomas Tegg; 1826, pp. 1–14.
11. Liston R. Injuries and Diseases of the Genito-Urinary Organs. In *Practical Surgery*. London: John Churchill; 1846, pp. 444–526.

13 Surgical Pain – Local Anaesthesia: James Moore (1762–1860)

INTRODUCTION

James Moore was born into a well-to-do family in Glasgow on 21 December 1762. His father was a physician, and his mother was the daughter of a professor of divinity at Glasgow University. He studied medicine in Edinburgh and London. He also served as an army medical officer in the American War of Independence [1]. In 1784, the year he became a member of the Surgeons' Company of London, he wrote a short book with the title 'A Method of Preventing or Diminishing Pain in Several Operations of Surgery' [2].

A New Method of Inducing Loss of Sensibility

This book was ignored for more than two centuries, until in 2024 two publications, one a paper and another a web page, expressed interest in the work of James Moore [3, 4]. Nonetheless, at the time, the book did not go unnoticed, being mentioned in the surgical textbooks of both James Latta [5] and Benjamin Bell [6]. Nonetheless, the method never became widely accepted, and the reasons for this deserve attention.

Moore's Technique of Local Anaesthesia Using Compression

For fifteen pages, Moore speculates on surgeons, humanity, cruelty, and the need for pain relief during operations. It is easy to find his speculations naïve and even rather inappropriate for one who had so limited experience of the profession he analysed. Nonetheless, his logic is clear and simple. He noted that sensation is communicated via the nerves. He also noted that sitting in certain positions could produce numbness and tingling in the leg. He observed that these positions imposed pressure on the sciatic nerve. Thus, he queried whether pressure could be used to dampen the sensibility of the nerves during amputation. His discussion is a fine example of how real anatomy had penetrated medical education. Having decided on the location where pressure should be applied (over the sciatic and femoral nerves), he experimented on himself in an attempt to numb one of his legs. At first, this was unsuccessful until he remembered that the numbness arising from an uncomfortable sitting position took time to develop. He soon found that he became aware of the numbness after about a quarter of an hour of compression.

DOI: 10.1201/9781003748816-13

Having discovered how to induce numbness, he then speculated on the underlying mechanism. He mentioned the animal spirits, which, according to humoural physiology, were supposed to transmit information in the nerves. Like Daniel Turner before him (see Chapter 7), he queried their existence. He added to Turner's speculations with the following impressive text.

> *The idea that a certain fluid, which has been distinguished by the name of animal spirits, flows in the nerves, and that it is by the means this fluid and its free egress and regress to and from the brain, that motion and sensibility depend, has been adopted by physiologists of the greatest eminence. Yet as this fluid has never been made evident to the senses, but has baffled the researches of the most dexterous anatomists, its existence can be considered as no more than a mere hypothesis, and of course it is possible that no such fluid does exist. On the supposition of such a fluid, it might naturally be expected, that upon compressing the nerves in the manner above described, the numbness and loss of voluntary motion of the parts below the compression would take place instantly; whereas, we find, that they happen in a very gradual manner, and are not complete till after a considerable time. Which seems rather to favour the suspicion many entertain, that no such fluid as the animal spirits does exist, but that the brain and nerves perform their functions by some other means, which nobody has ever yet been able to discover or explain [2].*

The anatomical relationships that Moore had to consider were as follows. A tourniquet applied to a limb compresses arteries, veins, and nerves, amongst other structures. The arteries and veins of the leg enter the limb at the front. The major nerves enter the limb at the front and at the back. At the front the artery, nerve and vein lie side by side, with the vein being the innermost and the nerve the outermost. The aim of Moore's treatment was to compress only the nerves. However, because there are multiple smaller arteries which enter the leg independently of the major vessels, compressing the artery could be accepted because these lesser arteries would maintain the blood supply. Experience had shown, in operations on aneurysms, that occlusion of the major artery could be tolerated for up to a couple of hours. Occlusion of the vein did not worry Dr Moore, although his instrument was designed to avoid it. It is illustrated in Figure 13.1. It should be applied so that the pad at the back was placed over the sciatic nerve. The pad at the front was placed over the femoral nerve, which lay just external to the easily palpable artery. However, there is another nerve entering the thigh nearer to the midline, and it would not be included in the pressure. This nerve supplied sensation to parts of the thigh, which would remain sensitive to pain. This meant that the compression could only be used for amputations below the knee.

As outlined above, Moore had worked out the details of his instrument by applying it to himself until he was convinced of its effectiveness. The next stage was to try it on a patient, and no less a person than John Hunter agreed to provide a patient who needed a below-the-knee amputation. The operation was pain-free to all intents, which is remarkable. The effectiveness of the compression was highlighted when the instrument was removed, and a vein started to bleed. This was ligated, and the patient stated that the pain of that ligation exceeded any discomfort he had experienced during the amputation. This experience demonstrated that the technique could work. Further research would be needed to determine its clinical reliability.

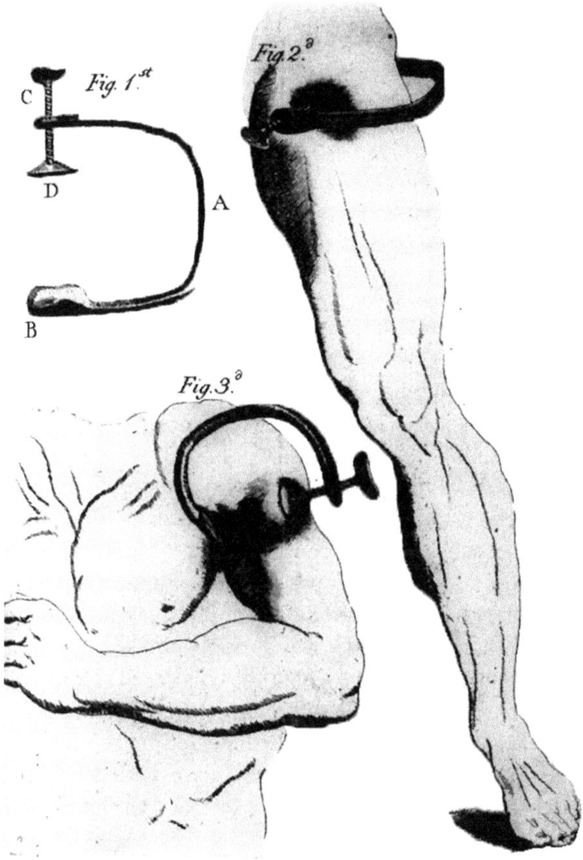

FIGURE 13.1 James Moore's compression device.

The image is taken from Moore's book but has been edited to improve clarity.

FURTHER DEVELOPMENTS

Both James Latta [5] and Benjamin Bell [6] applauded Moore for his device but were worried about its practical application, as both were concerned that compression of the vein could lead to an intolerable increase in venous pressure, which in turn could cause a burst vein. Both surgeons noted that Moore had reacted to this criticism by suggesting that the vein could be drained. Both men felt that this was an unsatisfactory solution. They would not accept the apparatus until they could be certain that the veins were not compressed.

Moore's book was noticed by others. Sir James Simpson, who introduced chloroform as an alternative to ether anaesthesia, commented on it in a paper on local anaesthesia. He noted the method and the success of the Hunter patient, and remarked that the method was well worthy of study [7]. Further comment is found in a booklet by the surgeon William Griffin, published in 1826. Griffin wrote:

It was imagined, not long since, by Dr Moore of London, that even the pain of the knife might be eluded by making compression on the nerve, supplying the diseased limb with sensibility, and thus preventing the transmission of the impression to the brain. The experiment was tried both in France and England; but though M. Baron Percy appears not to think unfavourably of it, the plan seems eventually to have fallen into disrepute. Patients under amputation still exhibited considerable variety in the apparent degree of suffering; yet as they had not experienced the pain of amputation without compression, it was excessively difficult to estimate the comparative merits of the two modes. A patient was at length operated on in St. Bartholomew's Hospital, who had formerly had a limb amputated in the usual manner; but he complained loudly of the numbness produced by the compression, and, so far from conceiving his suffering alleviated, declared that lie would much rather have the operation performed without it [8].

TOURNIQUETS AND SENSIBILITY

There is a certain amount of information related to compression and limb sensibility in the literature. However, this does not concern a specially designed instrument for that purpose, but rather addresses the consequences of applying tourniquets, which compress the entire limb. A recent paper analyses the development of the use of tourniquets for haemostasis. It laments the lack of clear-cut knowledge about the method's history and about the optimal way to apply compression [9]. It would seem that one of the earliest mentions of the technique concerned soldiers of Alexander the Great who were bitten by snakes following the Battle of Hydaspes in the valley of the Indus River in 326 BC. Alexander commandeered local Hindu physicians, who applied tourniquets to the bitten soldiers [9]. This experience was not transferred into Greek and subsequently Roman practice, so that tourniquets were unknown in ancient Rome.

In the European literature, the first mention of using a tourniquet to reduce sensibility is to be found in the writings of Henri de Mondeville:

Encircle the limb with two tightly wrapped cords or towels. Place one just below the joint and the other on the healthy side of the site of the amputation. Two aides must grasp the limb securely, above and below, to enable the surgeon to do his work in a stable field. The tight bindings will reduce the patient's sensibility [10].

Two hundred years later, Paré described the use of ligatures during the amputation of limbs. He writes:

Lastly there is a triple use of Ligatures in amputation of members, as arms and legs. The first to draw and hold upwards the skin and muscles lying under it, that the operation being performed; they may, by their falling down again, cover the ends of the cut-off bones; and so by that means help forwards the agglutination and cicatrization; and when it is healed up, cause the lame member to move more freely, and with lesse pain; and also to performe the former actions, this, as it were, cushion or boulster of musculous flesh lying thereunder. The second is, they hinder the bleeding by pressing together the veins and arteries. The third is, they by strait binding intercept the free passage of the animall spirits and so deprive the part which lyes thereunder of the sense of feeling, by making it, as it were, stupid or num [11].

James Yonge (1646/47 to 1721) was a British Royal Naval Surgeon from Plymouth. He was quite a prolific author and, in a book promoting the virtues of oil of turpentine there is a note on compression affecting the pain suffered during amputation. He wrote:

> *Sir, I hope it will not be altogether impertinent, if I here take occasion to recommend to the young Practitioner, one way of Ligature very useful in Amputations, especially above the Knee; that is to say, a wadd of hard linnen cloth, or the like, inside the Thigh a little below the Inguen, then passing a Towel round: the member; knit the ends of it together, and with a Battoon, a Bedstaff, or the like; twist it, till it compress the Wadd or Boulster so very strait on the crural Vessel, that (the circulation being stopped in them), their bleeding when divided by the Excision, shall be scarce large enough to let him see where to apply his Restrictives, nor shall the pain of that Operation be comparable to what it would be, were not the member nummed by the Compress [12].*

Heister also used the same technique:

> *Things being thus far advanced the Surgeon, who should have a Napkin before him, to wipe his Hands when there may be occasion, proceeds to fix the Tourniquet moderately tight about the Patient's Arm in the manner we before directed by which means the brachial Artery will be compressed, so as to prevent any profuse Haemorrhage; and the Nerve being also a Partaker of the same Stricture, will make the Patient less sensible of the Pain from the Operation [13].*

CONCLUSIONS

James Moore's apparatus to compress the nerves was a bold and sensible attempt to avoid the agony of surgery. However, from the available evidence, it would seem that its effects were inconsistent. It is not difficult to imagine that applying the apparatus in precisely the correct location was not easy and was conceivably time-consuming. In addition, variations in body shape and degree of obesity would add to the problems. There is also no explanation of how the pad over the sciatic nerve was maintained in position when the patient was lying supine. The use of the implement is described only for two patients, one of whom disliked its effects. The more general matter of reducing pain sensibility by generalized compression of a limb had been observed since the thirteenth century; a fact of which Moore made no mention.

REFERENCES

1. Moore J. *Oxford Dictionary of National Biography*. Oxford: Oxford University Press; 2004.
2. Moore J. *A Method of Preventing or diminishing Pain in Several Operations of Surgery*. London: T. Cadell; 1784.
3. Wildsmith J. James (Carrick) Moore (1763–1860*): Another (Scottish) Local Anaesthetic Hero. *Journal of the Royal College of Physicians of Edinburgh*. 2024; 54(4): 335–9.
4. Parker J. *To Conquer Pain: A Man Ahead of His Time and the Edinburgh Connections*. 2024. Available from: https://surgeonshallmuseums.wordpress.com/2024/10/04/to-conquer-pain-a-man-ahead-of-his-time-and-the-edinburgh-connections

5. Latta J. Of Diminishing the Pain of Chirurgical Operations. In *A Practical System of Surgery. II.* Edinburgh: G Mudie & Son; 1795, pp. 533–4.
6. Bell B. Of Preventing or Diminishing Pain in Chirurgical Operations. In *A System of Surgery. VII.* 6th ed. Edinburgh: Bell & Bradfute; 1796, pp. 393–7.
7. Simpson JY. Local Anæsthesia. *London Medical Gazette.* 1848 (March): 62–8.
8. Griffin W. *An Essay on the Nature of Pain.* Edinbugh: John Moir; 1826.
9. Kragh JF, Swan KG, Smith DC, Mabry RL, Blackbourne LH. Historical Review of Emergency Tourniquet Use to Stop Bleeding. *The American Journal of Surgery.* 2012; 203: 242–52.
10. De Mondeville H. Methods for Amputating Extremities and sawing Diseased Bones. In *Methods for Amputating Extremities and sawing Diseased Bones. The Surgery of Henri de Mondeville. II.* Bloomington, IN: XLibris; 2003, pp. 730–6.
11. Johnson T. Of the Uses for Which Ligatures Serve. In *The Workes of the Famous Chirurgion Ambroise Pare: Translated out of the Latine and Compared with the French.* London: Richard Cotes; 1649, p. 360.
12. Yonge J. *Account of the Many Admirable Vertues of Oleum Terebinthin.* London: J. Martyn; 1679.
13. Heister L. Amputation of the Hand, Humerus and Cubitus. In *A General System of Surgery in Three Parts. I.* London: W Innys; 1743, pp. 334–40.

14 Pain and Surgery – Conclusions

INTRODUCTION

In the modern English translation by T.A. Osbaldeston and R.P.A Wood, it is stated that Dioscorides actually used the Greek word anaesthesia, meaning insensitivity [1]. The first operation under ether was undertaken by William Thomas Green Morton (1819 to 1868) on 30 September 1846. This new process would obviously require a name, and Oliver Wendell Holmes the Elder (1809 to 1894), a renowned physician and scholar, provided the term anaesthesia. What made him choose this term remains uncertain. An older medical history book insists that the terms anaesthesia and anaesthetic were in common use throughout the eighteenth century [2]. Since Holmes was familiar with ancient Greek, it seems not unlikely that he had come across the word elsewhere, including in the work of Dioscorides from the first century AD. Nonetheless, his suggestion has become universally accepted. Developments since then have made the pain of surgery mostly a matter of historical interest. For most of the time prior to 1846, accounts of surgery and its problems were almost entirely restricted to the writings of surgeons. However, there have been a small number of accounts written by patients, and four of these follow. They demonstrate how the reaction to the pain of surgery reflected the personality, experience, and condition of the patient.

FOUR ACCOUNTS OF SURGERY WITHOUT ANAESTHESIA

Fanney Burney

The first case was the author Fanny Burney (1752–1840). She married a Frenchman in 1793, four years after the French Revolution. In 1802, he returned to France in an attempt to regain property he had lost during the troubled preceding years. In September 1811, Frances was diagnosed with cancer in her right breast and underwent a mastectomy, performed by Dominique-Jean Larrey, military surgeon to Napoleon. Despite the horror of the procedure, she lived another twenty-nine years, dying in 1840 at the age of eighty-seven. The following is a small extract from what she wrote of the experience.

> *When the dreadful steel was plunged into the breast – cutting through veins-arteries-flesh-nerves- I needed no injunction not to restrain my cries. I began a scream that lasted unintermittently during the whole time of the incision...Oh Heavens!-I then felt the knife racking against the breast bone – scraping it! This was performed while I yet remained in utterly speechless torture [3].*

DOI: 10.1201/9781003748816-14

George Young

An equally dramatic account is written by a twenty-five-year-old medical graduate called George Young, who in January 1843 underwent an amputation of an infected leg, which would otherwise have killed him. He left the following description of the experience.

> *I have recently read, with mingled sadness and surprise, the declarations of some surgeons that anaesthetics are needless luxuries, and that unendurable agony is the best of tonics. Those surgeons, I think, can scarcely have been patients of their brother surgeons....Of the agony it occasioned, I will say nothing. Suffering so great as I underwent cannot be expressed in words.... The particular pangs are now forgotten; but the black whirlwind of emotion, the horror of darkness, and the sense of desertion by God and man, bordering close upon despair, which swept through my mind and overwhelmed my heart, I can never forget, however gladly I would do so. From all this anguish I should of course have been saved had I been rendered insensible by ether or chloroform... before submitting to the operation [4].*

Apart from recording the soul-destroying extremity of the pain, this passage also provides a mention of a less-than-attractive characteristic found in some people in a position of authority, that pain can be beneficial.

Thomas Jackson

A third account is described by a sergeant wounded in battle on 8 March 1814, in the Netherlands at the Siege of Bergen-op-Zoom, a fortification held by the French in the south of that country. His unit surrendered in the evening of that day, and he became a wounded prisoner of the French. He survived for three days in the cold. Five times, his belongings were rummaged through by itinerant French soldiers or camp followers. Not only were his belongings stolen, but also whatever scraps of miserable bread had been distributed to the wounded soldiers. On the 10th of March, he finally met a surgeon who operated on him the following day, over three days after the injury. The leg was stinking. He describes the procedure as follows, starting with an introductory remark from the surgeon.

> *He said: "How do you feel, sergeant?" I said, "Sir, I feel very low and weak, but am anxious to have this stinking leg off." He, smiling, said "He was glad to hear such courage," and began to make preparation. "But sir," I said, "I feel myself in that feeble state, that I fear I shall sink under the operation, unless you will please give me some wine." He said "Well, you shall have some."*
>
> *So he gave some money to a bystander, to fetch me a bottle; but when he brought it, it was a Rhenish white wine and I did not like it: I said, "Let me have the red wine." He sent it back to be changed, and I had red wine. By this time they had got me fixed upon the end of a long barrack table, sitting upright, with my legs hanging down: a bason [sic] was brought for me to drink out of. I said, "Sir, let me have a good draught." He poured out nearly a pint, which I eagerly drank off. In an instant it wrought a wonderful effect, and raised up my spirits to an invincible courage. "Now, gentlemen," said I, "go*

> *on, if you please." The sergeant was preparing to blindfold me: "Oh, no;" I said, "I shall sit still, and see as well as the rest." One of the surgeons sat on a stool, to hold the leg steady; the second ripped up my trousers, and took down the stocking low enough; then he waited on the head surgeon. He, with a knife, much like that of a shoemaker's, took his place at my right hand (it being the right leg to be amputated), the tourniquet being placed painfully tight above the knee; he put his hand under the calf of the leg, and setting the edge of the knife on the shin bone, at one heavy, quick stroke, drew it round, till it met the shin bone again. All eyes were fixed on me, but I was too high spirited then to give way.*
>
> *Next, the surgeon, with his hand, forced up the flesh toward the knee, to make way for the saw. When the saw was applied, I found it extremely painful; it was worn out; it stuck in the way, as a bad saw would when sawing a green stick. I said, "Oh, sir, have you not a better saw?" He said, he was sorry he had not, as they were all worn out. The bone got through, the next thing to be done was still more painful – that of tying up the ligatures; then followed the drawing down of the flesh to cover the end of the bone, and tightly strapped there with strips of sticking plaster; after this, strongly bandaged: and thus ended the operation, which lasted about half an hour [5].*

This quotation is lengthy because it illustrates a very different reaction to the awful pain of surgery. Military training and the acceptance of pain as an unavoidable component of his job make this account far more accepting. It should, however, be remembered that the sergeant had chosen a military career, indicating at least that he was prepared for the discomfort such a career might force him to bear. The three accounts are powerful evidence of the importance of the personality of the patient and the circumstances of the procedure.

Artur Rubinstein

Finally, there is the experience of one of the world's most famous musicians when he was still a young man making his way. In 1907, the young pianist Artur Rubinstein had settled in Paris and given two concerts, which impressed people so much that Count Nicholas Potocki, a Polish compatriot who was also one of the richest men in Europe, became aware of him and invited him to stay in his country home for the summer. There, while fishing, he pricked his right index finger while removing a fish from the hook. A paronychia developed, and a doctor was called, who correctly advised surgery. There was no available anaesthetic, and time was of the essence. Rubinstein begged the doctor to operate as his career depended on keeping a normal finger. His account of the operation is as follows.

> *He pierced the very spot of the infection with a small silver stiletto and began to dig around inside the tip of my finger for a good minute or two, while I squirmed on my chair and shrieked at the top of my voice. The pain was indescribable.*
>
> *"This is the only way to get the pus out," the doctor said when I came to after a short spell of faintness.*
>
> *He tortured me three more times before the ordeal was over. Since he never asked me for a fee, I suppose he sent the bill to the Count [6].*

DIVERSE TOPICS

There are inevitably a number of components of a surgical treatment that may affect the pain of a treatment. The timing of surgery is one of these. Surgeons may wish to delay an operation to ensure that on the day of surgery, all relevant conditions are as optimal as possible. In painful conditions, any delay results in extending the duration of pain. This may make good surgical sense, as when delaying the drainage of an abscess until it has become fluctuant. However, the decisions of timing were often subjective and traditionally could include consideration of the time of year and the state of the planets; the importance of which is demonstrated by this text from Guy de Chauliac, concerning the origin of the Black Death

> *The General Cause was derived from the conjunction of the three superior planets, Saturn, Jupiter and Mars that had been preceded by another conjunction on March 24, 1345, in the 14th degree of Aquarius. Those great conjunctions, as I explained in my book on astrology, signified amazing, potent, and terrible things, such as changes in kings, appearances of prophets, and of great plagues [7].*

Another component of treatment that could be painful is the management of dressings. Pressure dressings called tents were popular through the ages, but Wiseman advocated avoiding them, for example, in the treatment of small wounds, as their use delayed healing and caused pain [8]. Moreover, Woodall advised against their use in the treatment of abscesses since their placement within an abscess cavity hindered drainage and hence healing [9].

The influences of astrology or dressings on the pain of treatment are not considered. Astrology is ignored because it is nonsense. The influence of dressings is ignored because the cause of pain is avoidable. In this book, the concern is solely with the pains of surgery, which cannot be avoided, including the cut of the knife, the heat of the cautery, and the manipulation of the tissues.

THE SPEED OF SURGERY

It is clear that shorter operations will, in general, produce less pain than longer procedures. This means also that the speed of the surgeon, prior to anaesthesia, was an important parameter affecting his reputation and impacting on his ability to acquire patients. On the other hand, speed carried with it risk. This is exemplified by the experience of Robert Liston (1794–1847), a surgeon so speedy that he could amputate a leg in under thirty seconds. However, the price of such speed was the occasional serious error [10]. An alternative approach was that of Ambroise Paré, who prized precision, gentleness, and accuracy above all else [11]. Both made substantial contributions to surgery. Another surgeon who was highly respected and who acquired great wealth was William Cheselden, who had the reputation of performing a lithotomy for bladder stone in under 30 seconds. Despite the importance of speed, there is really no data enabling a correlation between the speed of a surgeon and the quality of his results. Thus, while speed has been mentioned, it is also an aspect of the management of surgical pain which was not further analysed.

Finally, in view of the need to respect considerations of diversity, equality, and inclusion, it is necessary to comment that the pronoun 'he' is used throughout the book. A comment from a recent publication reads as follows:

> *Regulations for the practice of surgery were widely recognized and often barred women. In 1313, women were banned from the practice of surgery in Paris unless examined by a competent jury. Except for widows, who were allowed to assume the surgical practices of their late husbands during the 14th and 15th centuries, no other women were allowed to practise. In the 14th century, King Henry VIII was quoted as saying "No carpenter, smith, weaver or women shall practise surgery." Further, in 1540, he granted the charter for the Company of Barber Surgeons; women were barred. Women did, however, continue to practise during this time. They continued to practise without formal training or recognition in England and eventually North America for the next several centuries [12].*

Since women were barred from surgical practice and since those who nonetheless practiced left no record of their work, the people whose work can be discussed in the context of this book were all men. Hence, the choice of pronoun.

SUMMARIZATION

Accessible texts on the topic of surgery really begin with Hippocrates. From then on up to the end of the Middle Ages, pain would seem to have been an unavoidable component of daily life, with no means available for its relief. In the Christian world, this became less relevant as it was generally agreed that the health of the soul had a higher priority than the health of the body. Thus, while there were limited improvements in patient management through these centuries, they were limited. The major method of managing surgical pain was acceptance of the unavoidable, amplified by the impact of the surgeon's personality.

Following the Black Death and the ensuing disappearance of feudalism, the importance of every individual in the state increased, no matter their social standing. Improvements in pain management began to appear. In the sixteenth century, surgeons expressed a more humane attitude, none more than Ambroise Paré. Thereafter, opium was permitted to relieve the pain of illness and post-operative care. Vesalius' textbook of anatomy led to a much better understanding of the components of the body, which might be exposed to surgery. Then Harvey presented his book on the circulation of the blood, the first body blow to the nonsense humoral physiology which had survived since Hippocrates and Galen.

From the time of the Enlightenment, attempts were made to improve instruments and surgical technique to minimize patient suffering. From the end of the Enlightenment, the attempts at technical improvement became more profound and varied until 1846, when anaesthesia was invented, and the problem simply went away.

CONCLUSIONS

It seems fair from the material accumulated in this book to suggest that tolerance of pain has decreased over the centuries, especially since the nineteenth century, when effective measures for its alleviation became more and more available. Surgeons, like patients, are human and variable. Some behave in extreme fashions, but most are decent and well-motivated. I have met brilliant surgeons, stupid surgeons, and greedy surgeons. However, I have never met the sort of sadistic surgeons described in critical descriptions of the profession. Maybe they exist, but if they do, they are exceedingly rare. Certainly, constant contact with blood, the insides of human bodies, and the various unpleasant processes that affect them make surgeons inured to the natural reactions of those who do not have a similar experience. To conclude, no writer has encapsulated the problem of the pain of operations better than Celsus in ancient Rome in the first century AD.

> *Now a surgeon should be youthful or at any rate nearer youth than age; with a strong and steady hand which never trembles, and ready to use the left hand as well as the right; with vision sharp and clear, and spirit undaunted; filled with pity, so that he wishes to cure his patient, yet is not moved by his cries, to go too fast, or cut less than is necessary; but he does everything just as if the cries of pain cause him no emotion [13].*

REFERENCES

1. Dioscorides. *Dioscorides de Materia Medica*. Johannesburg: Ibidis Press; 2000.
2. Mettler CC. Nineteenth Century. In: Mettler FA, editor. *History of Medicine*. Philadelphia, PA: The Blakiston Company; 1947.
3. Porter R. Hospitals and Surgery. In *The Cambridge History of Medicine*. Cambridge, MA: Cambridge University Press; 2011, pp. 176–210.
4. Adler RE. *Such Stuff as Dreams are Made On: The Discovery of Anesthesia. Medical Firsts from Hippocrates to the Human Genome*. Hoboken, NJ: John Wiley and Sons; 2004, pp. 83–93.
5. Jackson T. *Narrative of the Eventful Life of Thomas Jackson*. Warwick: Helion & Company Limited; 2018.
6. Rubinstein A. *My Young Years*. New York: Knopf Doubleday; 1973.
7. de Chauliac G. Treatise II The Aposthems. In *Doctrine II Eight Chapters: Aposthems in Particular Places. The Major Surgery of Guy de Chauliac an English Translation.* Bloomington, IN: Xlibris Corporation; 2007, pp. 247–50.
8. Wiseman R. Of Wounds in General. In *Eight Chirurgical Treatises*. London: Walthoe, J et al.; 1734, pp. 39–62.
9. Woodall J. Of the Medicines, and Their Uses. In *The Surgions Mate*. London: Edward Griffin; 1617, p. 68.
10. Hawk AJ. ArtiFacts: Built for Speed—Robert Liston's Surgical Technique. *Clinical Orthopaedics and Related Research*. 2021; 479: 679–80.
11. Johnson T. *The Workes of the Famous Chirurgion Ambroise Pare: Translated out of the Latine and Compared with the French*. London: Richard Cotes; 1649.
12. Wirtzfield DA. The History of Women in Surgery. *Canadian Journal of Surgery*. 2009; 52(4): 317–20.
13. Celsus. Book VII, Proemium. In *De Medicina*. Cambridge, MA: Loeb Library, Harvard University Press; 1938, pp. 295–9.

Index

Pages in *italics* refer to figures, and pages followed by "n" refer to notes.

D

E

F

G

H

M

N

T

U

V

W

Y

Z

www.ingramcontent.com/pod-product-compliance
Ingram Content Group UK Ltd.
Pitfield, Milton Keynes, MK11 3LW, UK
UKHW020204200926
475702UK00004B/613

9781041253822